A PREGNANCY MEMOIR

UTTHARA UNNI NITHESH

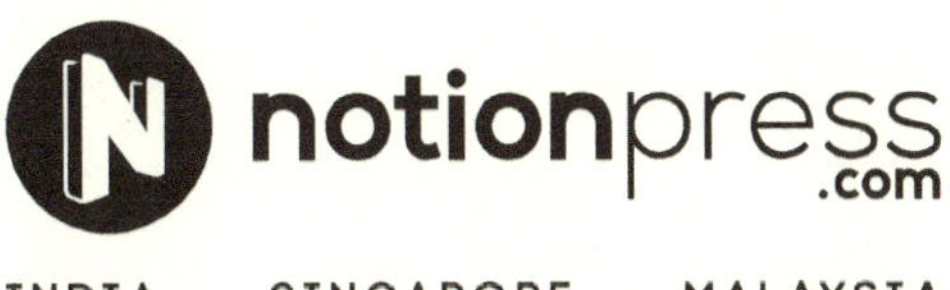

INDIA • SINGAPORE • MALAYSIA

ISBN 979-8-89233-777-9

CONTENTS

FOREWORD

It is a matter of great pleasure for me to write the foreword for this book "A Pregnancy Memoir".

I congratulate Mrs. Utthara Unni Nithesh from the depth of my heart for brilliantly depicting her journey to motherhood, mixing both scientific facts and locally popular myths.

This book is a wonderful piece of literature, emphasising the role of a healthy lifestyle and physical fitness, especially dancing, in achieving a successful pregnancy outcome.

With best wishes and warmest regards,

Dr. Susan John
Senior Consultant Gynaecologist &
Laparoscopic Surgeon
Ernakulam Medical Centre, Kochi

"Every story has a beautiful or sad ending. But this story ends with a beautiful beginning."

PROLOGUE

I have always loved writing but I still don't think I can call myself a writer. I did not believe I'd write a book and pregnancy was the last topic I thought I'd choose. My pregnancy was not a cakewalk if you are wondering how I wrote an entire book. Well, fortunately, it wasn't a rocky road either. This book started as a simple journal and my inquisitiveness led me to read, research and understand furthermore on this topic.

I was always a health freak. I started exercising at the age of sixteen when I had dreams of taking up acting and modelling as a career and wanted to maintain a Barbie figure. But things don't always work out the way you wish. I moved to Chennai for my college. I graduated with B.Sc. Visual Communication and mastered in M.A. Communication. Meanwhile, I developed an interest in dance which my mom tried to instil in me since my childhood. I graduated with B.F.A. Bharatanāṭyam under the special guidance of Padma Bhūṣaṇ Dr. Padma Subrahmanyam and mastered in M.A. Bharatanāṭyam. I did not fall in love with dance as crazily as I did with cinema but before I knew it I was married to dance. Well, if there's an option I'd still continue to have an affair with cinema, my first love.

I became a performing artist and I took up this beautiful art of teaching. Eventually, I fell in love with what I was doing. Dance has made me who I am. It is a journey towards your deeper self. It has given me a reputation in the society, it pays my bills and keeps me mentally sane and physically fit. Dance is the reason that wakes me up every single day.

I was not an active child. I was quiet and enjoyed my very own company in the world of storybooks and dolls. I'd make sure to come up with an excuse on sports days or other physically tormenting days in school. I don't remember playing run-around games or ball games much in my childhood either. I always preferred silent imaginative games in my bedroom rather than sunny outdoor games.

I booked myself for a trip to Bali at the age of twenty-five. It was an adventure trip for a group of solo travellers who belonged to the same age group. That was one of the most spontaneous things I had ever done in my life. I even got myself a tattoo from Bali. A star tattoo that will remind me that I will always be a star, no matter what. Since it was an adventure trip, we had several activities like surfing, snorkelling, scuba diving, trekking etc. I realised I was healthier and stronger than many twenty-five-year-olds when I could hike up a mountain on the second day of my menstrual cycle without any discomfort. I realised my balance on a surfboard was smoother than many although I had never seen a surfboard in my life.

If dance was not a part of my life I wouldn't have become such an active person. I'd probably be suffering from unhealthy conditions like PCOD or psychological issues which are caused mainly due to lack of exercise. A typical Bharatanāṭyam recital would be 1.5 hours long. You need to dance every day for at least two hours to gain that stamina to perform ceaselessly. Strength training is necessary to get stronger and enough stretches are needed to decrease the risk of injuries. To maintain a life that involves 3-4 hours of physical work - a healthy diet, sufficient water intake and quality hours of sleep are a must. So it's not just dance; one thing leads to another and it's all interconnected.

I have no medical background, I'm not a certified nutritionist and I'm not an expert in fitness training. This book is a casual read about my journey into motherhood and my simple findings from my personal experience evaluated and approved by doctors. Half of this book was written during my pregnancy and half during the first two months postpartum. And so this book is wholeheartedly dedicated to the wonderful miracle that blossomed in my womb - My daughter - Dheemahee.

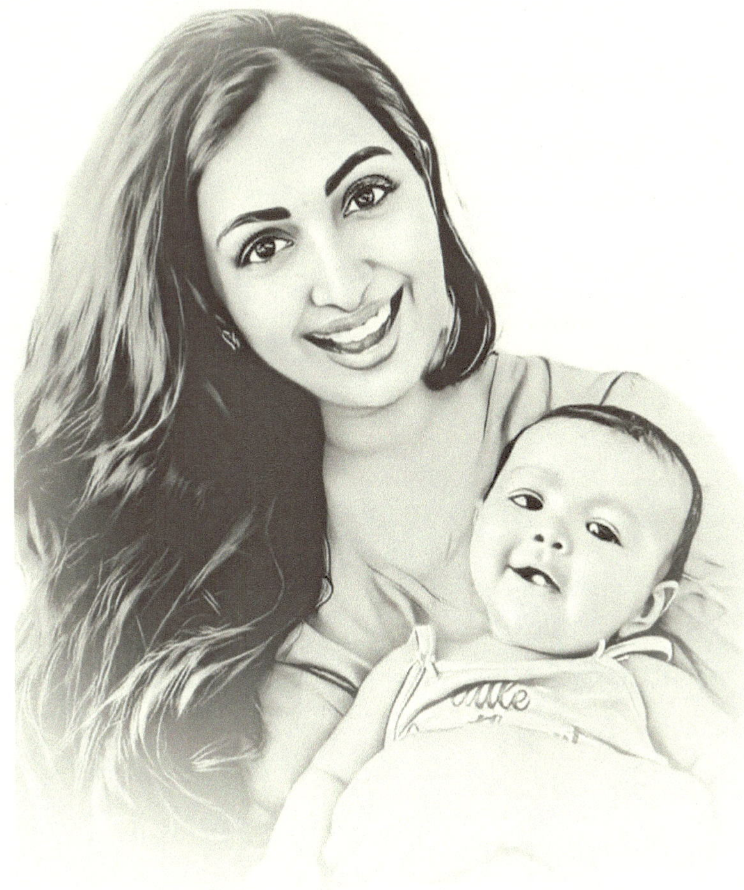

Thank you for choosing this book and I hope I don't let you down.

Firsts are always special. But I don't think anything in the world can be more special than seeing a life come to fruition within you. The human body is designed to be capable of creating such a marvel and I'm just beginning to experience this beautiful journey - My first pregnancy.

I was always ready to be a mom. I loved playing mom games as a child - feeding my dolls, bathing them, dressing them up and putting them to sleep. I'd wear my mom's saree, carry her handbag and act like an adult. We were given fake money so that we could play like we had bills to pay and work to attend. With a tiny kitchen set, it was another realm altogether. I wanted long hair like my mom. My friends and I would use mom's shawls to cover the sides of the dining table and sit underneath, believing that it was our home and play with our Barbie dolls all day long.

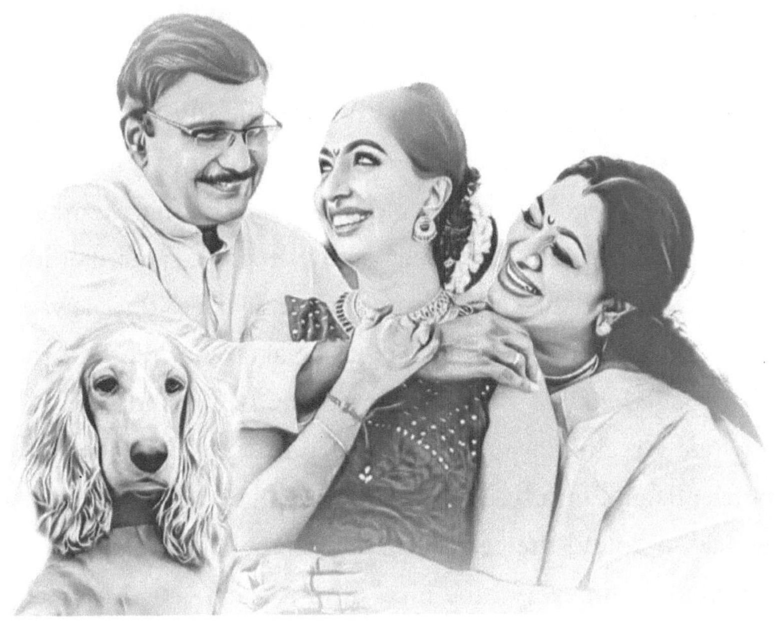

But adulting was nothing like the princess stories we had heard. It was a slap on the face. Finding love wasn't easy, getting married wasn't facile. I wanted to find the right person, get married happily and then begin my motherhood on a peaceful and safe mental space because I believe that good human beings are children raised in pleasant environments. I believe that kids need to grow up in families that do not conduct wars. My childhood was a mix of arts and academics, glitter and grey, calm and chaos. My parents were like black and white; hence I'm a mix of all. My knowledgeable, well-read, wise dad's ideologies were the opposite of that of the artistic glam queen that my mom was. I was fortunate to have grown up in a heavenly abode - My mom, dad and me - and of course our important four-legged family members - Chilli and Momo - our doggos.

It took almost a year for me and my husband to understand how this relationship worked. Nithesh and I met on a matrimony website which was created and handled by my mother. I did not believe in finding love through an online portal. Finding your better half was not something to be done like shopping for clothes online. But to everyone's surprise, we clicked. We went on dates; Nithesh came home, met my parents, my parents met his family and before I had any choice, we were engaged. The photographs by Design Ads were so dreamy and gorgeous that I couldn't resist posting them. Nithesh proposed to me by tying silver bells on my feet as a symbol of love and a promise to keep dance alive throughout our lives. The news of this unique proposal idea went viral all over social media. We were then the famous engaged couple who were in vogue. It was indeed a fairytale night where I recited a poem for him and he spoke so graciously to all my friends and family. My parents were elated as if in the seventh heaven having found the perfect match for their only daughter. It was all "sugar, spice and everything nice" until it wasn't.

Then started a war! We were poles apart different and so we had arguments about anything and everything under the sun. Thanks to COVID-19 which bombarded out of nowhere to save me from this trap called Marriage. It gave us more than a year of courtship and we had the time to fight all the fights in the world before we tied the knot. Nithesh is a businessman and Managing Director of UTiZ Global Ventures & UTiZ Resource Management.

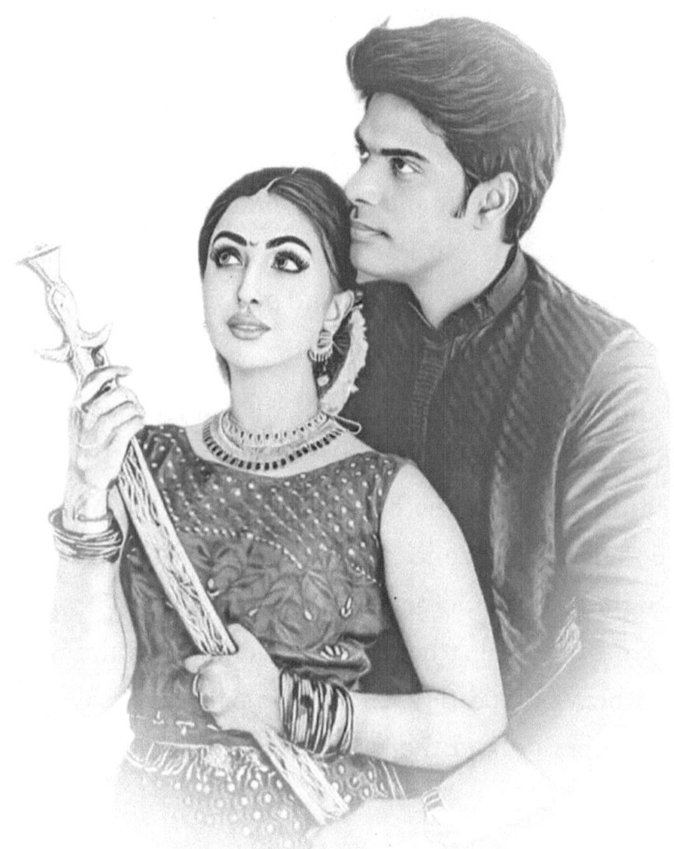

Once Nithesh and I started having an understanding of each other's moods and tantrums, we started getting along in a much more peaceful manner. As our relationship matured, we decided it was time to welcome a new member into our family. We started trying for a baby.

We had planned for a trip to Europe in September 2022. I had performances in Prague and Germany and we combined it with a holiday to Budapest, Austria and Switzerland. We both wanted to conceive in Switzerland so that years later we would have a story to tell. We could conceive a Swiss baby like Snow White - *"Her hair as black as ebony, her lips as red as rose"*. I think all women secretly wish to have a girl but then end up loving our boys more. Strange! Maybe I will answer that one day. Before the trip, I started taking folic acid and vitamin D tablets as suggested by my gynaecologist - Dr. Susan John (DGO, DNB, FRCOG) from EMC hospital who magically cured my period pain last year stating the reason was endometriosis. I did not even drink much of the famous Swiss wine or German beer during the trip. September 19th is Nithesh's birthday and October 14th is mine. We wanted to conceive on his and find out on my date. As a storyteller, I like to make everything dramatic.

After returning to India, I felt like I had all sorts of symptoms - a sudden common cold, tender breasts, heartburn at night, lethargy, eye twitching etc. With the help of the internet at our fingertips we tend to google all our concerns and queries. For all the questions I asked, google said I could be pregnant until I saw a drop of blood on 6th October. I still didn't believe it. I woke up in the middle of the night with heavy blood flow and severe pain and realised that I had to accept my period and that we weren't having a Swiss baby. I was downhearted.

My 30th birthday was arriving on the 14th of October and Nithesh was in Mumbai for work. So we decided to celebrate it there. A week before I heard that my grandmother's cousin Indramani Ammuma passed away. According to the Hindu tradition, we believe that when a soul passes away, the same soul is reborn in the family within the next year. The birthday night and the next night were party-hard nights where Nithesh wanted me to relive my twenties. I finally finished my Mumbai Diaries script - a movie script I had been working on for some time. As the baby planning didn't work out in the first month, we decided to move ahead with our movie plans. It's been a long break after my last directorial - the short film - Paw Prints. I decided to make a movie this year and started having discussions with production houses.

We went to Kovalam in the first week of November. Nithesh had a few meetings in Trivandrum and I thought I would sit in the room and work on editing my script. We stayed in Kovalam Leela to enjoy a day off and then drove back to Cochin. We don't know if we conceived in ITC Maratta in Mumbai or The Leela Palace in Kovalam, but we tested pregnancy positive on 8th November 2022.

I somehow had a gut feeling that I was going to be pregnant but it came as a huge surprise to Nithesh. He was flabbergasted and got very emotional. Tears rolled down his cheeks as the two red lines appeared on the test kit while we sat on our bed and eagerly waited. We immediately called up Dr. Susan who insisted on getting a few blood tests done. After a day we got our results and went to the hospital. We came back and told Amma and Acha who were more elated than ever. We video-called Mummy (Mother-in-law) to give the news and happiness filled her. After a few days, we had our first scan. It was too early to detect the heartbeat so we had to wait for a few more days to confirm the healthy pregnancy.

On 28th November we had our next scan and the heartbeat was confirmed. It felt like watching a miracle blossom - To see another life bloom inside. We saw a graphical twinkling on the monitor and we could hear the tiny heart sound like galloping horses. We both had teary eyes as we looked at the ultrasound monitor.

It was Chinnuka's (Samyuktha Varma) birthday, so we called Prabha (Valyamma), Chinnuka and Mālukka (Cousin) to give them the news. Then slowly our friends, extended family and my students heard the news. Everyone was happy and excited.

THE NĀGAS

The practice of snake worship in Sanāthana Dharma dates back to several centuries. Sarpa Prīti, Sarpa Pūjā etc. are performed to keep the snakes happy. Why is this being done? What is the significance or relevance of this worship in today's world?

The conception of a human embryo starts with the merging of a sperm and an egg. Out of thousands of sperm, only a single one gets to merge with the egg. The shape of this sperm resembles that of a snake. It has a head and a tail. This process of merging is called fertilisation.

The new cell that is formed from the sperm and egg is called the zygote. The zygote contains a unique DNA code (Deoxyribo Nucleic Acid) by taking chromosomes from both parents. Twenty-three chromosomes from the mother and twenty-three from the father are taken. When that child has a baby, the baby will contain eleven and a half chromosomes from his/her grandparents. This process continues for about eight hundred years until thirty-two generations are born for the last hereditary chromosome to become extinct. The root cause for all this is the DNA. The DNA decides the colour of the eyes, the shape and size of the body and many other factors. The DNA molecule is in the shape of two snakes mating with each other.

The fertilised egg stays in the fallopian tube for about three to four days but within the first twenty-four hours, it starts dividing into many cells and finally moves slowly through the fallopian tube to the uterus. As it multiplies, it is called a blastocyst. The next job is to attach itself to the lining of the uterus. This process is called implantation. Now it can be called an embryo.

At this point, a home pregnancy test could show positive results. The embryo is also in the shape of a snake. The placenta becomes its home. The embryo grows and starts forming eyes and ears. Arms and legs also start to form. By around the 10th week, the embryo becomes known as a foetus and that's what doctors call them until birth.

Every human being begins their life in the shape of a snake. The symbol of medical science is two snakes on a pillar. What makes a human complete is the nervous system. The nervous system's structure is also that of a snake - a head that is the brain and a tail that is the spine.

Therefore the sacred worship of Nāgas in Hinduism is not about worshiping snakes as Gods. It is about worshipping the consciousness of human beings and the existence of heredity.

YOGIC SYMBOLISM OF SNAKES

The Kundalini, the latent primordial energy of the universe, is believed to lie dormant at the base of the human spine. This is said to be in the shape of a coiled serpent. When this energy is awakened by yogic practices, it ascends, passing through six spiritual centres or chakras, until it reaches the top of the head. This point is considered the thousand-petalled chakra of total awareness and spiritual realisation. This energy that animates the universe is always represented as a serpent.

HCG

This is the first and most significant test done on pregnant women to check many parameters. hCG or Human Chorionic Gonadotropin is often known as the pregnancy hormone as it is a hormone produced by the placenta. hCG levels can be detected through blood tests about eleven days after conception and fourteen days through urine tests. A hCG level less than 5 mlU/mL is considered negative for pregnancy and anything above 25 mlU/mL is considered positive for pregnancy. Anything in between is a grey area and may need to be tested again. hCG number is supposed to double in 48 hours. However, an ultrasound should be able to confirm the findings. Low hCG may indicate possibilities for miscarriage, ectopic pregnancies etc. and high level may indicate multiple pregnancies or certain types of diseases. The Last Menstrual Period (LMP) is an important date to remember to calculate the age of the foetus. In most cases, hCG and ultrasound confirm the Expected Delivery Date (EDD).

ULTRASOUND

Ultrasound or USG (Ultrasonography) is an imaging method that uses sound waves to produce images of structures within the body. Commonly referred to as a scan, it can provide valuable information for diagnosing the baby's health conditions and development. Ultrasound is an important part of pregnancy. It is special as it is the first time couples get to "see" their baby. The first ultrasound is done during 6-12 weeks to know that the implantation has occurred at the right place and to monitor the heart rate of the foetus. Anomaly scan, also known as mid-pregnancy scan is done between 18-21 weeks to screen the baby's development in detail. Rare conditions like spina bifida, exomphalos, anencephaly and many others can be found and the doctor may suggest treatment options. In the third trimester, a final scan will confirm the position of the foetus to proceed with plans for delivery. The number of scans and the intervals at which they are done can also vary depending on the doctor and the mother's health.

There are two types of ultrasound which are commonly used-

- Transabdominal ultrasound - This is performed by moving the transducer across the belly. The patient is asked to drink water and make the bladder full as sound waves move easily to get a better picture.
- Transvaginal ultrasound - This is done by inserting the transducer into the birth canal. Don't worry it is not a painful procedure.

In rare cases, doppler ultrasound, 3D ultrasound or 4D ultrasound are used.

WHAT YOU NEED TO KNOW BEFORE GETTING PREGNANT

The clock ticks differently for each woman. While some are in a hurry to get married, get pregnant and settle down in life, some want to grow in their careers, travel the world and pause the pregnancy for a while.

However, a healthy lifestyle choice is important to receive positive outcomes. Everyone talks about what to eat and what not to eat during pregnancy. Everyone advises on exercise and activities during pregnancy. But no one talks about the importance of maintaining a healthy lifestyle months or years before planning to conceive. A woman's pre-pregnancy health matters in how easy things can be at a later stage.

Obesity, PCOD, Thyroid etc. are various ailments that are now extremely common among the youth. This is mainly due to the lifestyle and could cause major hindrance to conception.

A healthy diet, good exercise and a healthy lifestyle can not only help in conceiving or developing a healthy baby, it also helps in recovering and regaining the health and body to its previous form.

FOOD

What a person eats is directly or inversely proportional to how a person feels. Or vice versa. We all say that food is an emotion. Some people can hog and enjoy a meal wholeheartedly only if they are truly happy and at peace with their thoughts and surroundings. But for some, it's the other way. Some people hog when they are upset. For e.g. there's stress eating or sometimes anxiety eating and so many other things. The food one eats can also play a very vital role in keeping their mood intact. There's absolutely nothing to be ashamed of admitting that you are going through an emotional rough patch. Certain vitamin deficiencies can cause certain illnesses. Similarly, certain nutritional deficiencies can cause a wide variety of mood swings. Hormonal imbalances can be a major cause. The problem a lot of times is within your body and not the actual problem you are stressing on. Good food can help you keep your hormones balanced. Hormones decide your sex drive, fertility and how easily you can get pregnant or how fast you can shed the pregnancy weight. Regulating your blood sugar levels and improving insulin sensitivity will increase your chances of getting pregnant.

Therefore the first thing to do is to avoid packaged foods, hotel food and alcohol a few months or a year before trying to get pregnant. Quit smoking if you have a habit. Try to eat freshly cooked home food; not food that's been in the fridge for two days. These minute changes can sometimes work like magic.

EXERCISE

Do you know what is the one thing that can be more dangerous than drinking or smoking? Sitting! Sitting for long hours. It's a silent killer. We don't realise the amount of time we spend sitting. Sitting on the bed, sitting at your office desk, sitting in the car seat, sitting on a sofa and watching TV. Sitting or not moving your body can cause more hazardous effects on your body than you may imagine. One must have heard that bike riders lose sperm mobility and fertility due to the heat generated in the genital area from the bike's engine. Similarly many of us today are exposed to urinary infections and itching in the genital area due to the heat generated from long hours of just sitting. What we need to do is move around as and when possible.

Research says that just fifteen minutes of exercise a day can reduce the risk of heart attacks. But fifteen minutes out of twenty-four hours is still a very small amount of time. An increased amount of time dedicated to exercise can help with obesity, thyroid and PCOD - the main hindrances to getting pregnant. Exercise helps in regulating blood sugar levels which in turn improves your mental well-being, sex drive and egg/sperm quality. Just ten days of not exercising can double the amount of insulin in your body. A little effort from your end can show drastic changes in insulin sensitivity and it continues to stay strong for the next seventy-two hours. Blood sugar tests are done on pregnant women to check their chances of gestational diabetes. So forget the old concept of "eating for two" or enjoying the most of your pregnancy by hogging everything you crave for.

More exercise means less fat and more muscle mass. It is important to strengthen your muscles because more muscle mass means reduced insulin resistance and that makes way for better implantation of the foetus, less risk of gestational diabetes and faster fat burning and recovery post-delivery. When the muscles are stronger, the cells of the body can easily pick sugar from the blood stream and this helps to lower the blood sugar levels. During pregnancy, the body will reduce insulin sensitivity to make more nutrients for the foetus. Without strong muscles, the body will have a tough time adjusting to this change. That's why a lot of women with no history of diabetes develop gestational diabetes during pregnancy. Therefore, it is important to stay fit and healthy before, during and after pregnancy.

LIFESTYLE

The way you live your life decides the way your life is going to pay you back. Are you an early bird or a night owl? Are you a person who prefers home food over Zomato and Swiggy? Do you like to spend your nights reading and chilling at home or do you party hard every night till dawn? These little things speak volumes of who you are as a person. Try to bring in small changes to your lifestyle by making healthier choices.

The 1% rule by James Clear is that if you get 1% better each day then by the end of your time you become 37% better. Conversely, if you get 1% worse, you will get 37% worse. 1% may be such a small change that it may not even be noticeable but in the long run, it is going to make a lot of difference.

Stress and sleep are interconnected and interdependent. We are living in a busy world where overworking is considered as the new "Cool". A stressed-out body and brain means lesser quality sleep. Poor sleep reduces your health, brings an imbalance in your hormones, reduces chances of good sex and lowers the chances of a healthy pregnancy. An overworked body requires rest and sleep to recover. One needs to find that work-life balance. A little bit of compromise on your career growth is required if you feel it's taking a toll on your health.

THE TWO MINUTE RULE

When you're trying to build a new habit, it's not easy to start too big. When you think about the change you want to make, your excitement and motivation can convince you to do too much, too soon. But doing too much all of a sudden can drain you and make you lose interest before you realise it. Always try to sustain the interest, no matter what.

The two-minute rule says that your new habit should be something that takes just two minutes. For example, just walking up to your dance room, opening your laptop, and putting on your running shoes. These are things that don't require effort. Maybe just going to your dancing space and doing one Adavu (Step) should be your goal. Dancing for 3 hours should not be your initial goal. It will make you hate the dance and hate yourself for not meeting your goals. So start small and enjoy the process of making it a daily habit. Make it feel simple, psychologically. Everything else will simply fall into place.

POLLUTION

Air pollution can harm lung development by causing low birth weight, pre-term birth or improper immune system development. Air pollution to an extent can be controlled by personal lifestyle choices, for e.g. smoking. But other factors are not in our control. Pollution during the prenatal period may interfere with organ development or lead to organogenesis.

Anything that makes us sick reduces our ability to conceive. Like insulin resistance, air pollution also reduces the body's ability to pick nutrients from the blood. Moving to a city with less traffic and pollution or staying indoors etc. when you are trying to conceive could be more beneficial and may result in a healthier pregnancy.

YOUR PARTNER

The sexist world makes it feel like pregnancy is the sole responsibility of a woman. No, just like it takes two hands to clap, the health and lifestyle of your partner are equally important. It doesn't work when one person eats healthy, works out and sleeps right. Male fertility improves when the men make healthier choices. It leads to the production of better quality sperm which leads to better sex and easier conception. The mental and physical support from your partner is not just enough until conception, it is needed during the period of gestation and postpartum. Remember that a healthy baby needs a healthy mamma and for that, she needs a supportive dadda.

It is important to have a healthy relationship. Not just with your partner or friends, but with everything you do in your daily life. It is important to be on good terms with your food, your thoughts, your body, and your work. It is important to accept them and cherish them. There are days when I absolutely hate the idea of dancing, there are days when I can't get out of bed, there are days when I'm not excited about my 6 AM classes, there are days when I hate to dress up and there are days when I want to eat just pure junk food. We need to find that balance between pushing hard to be the best and not hating ourselves for not meeting our goals. We can't be our 100% on every single day. Understanding that it's okay to let loose on certain days and still trying to be your best could build a healthier relationship with yourself. Understanding that as humans we will have our ups and downs make us less prone to self-blaming

and guilt-tripping. Have a healthy relationship with your food. Know what you eat, know the ingredients and what it does to your body. Do things with your heart and do listen to what your body is saying. Maintain a very healthy and clean relationship with your food, sleep, work, body and everything that you do. And before you know it, your body will reward you.

THE FIRST TRIMESTER

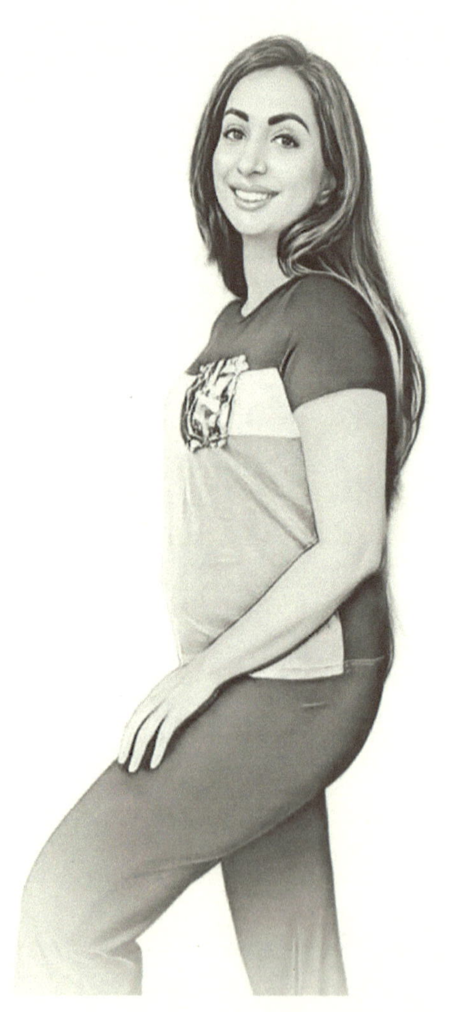

The first trimester was a disaster for me. I felt sick almost all the time from the 8th week to almost the 13th week. Nausea was beyond my endurance. I did not have any cravings, only aversions to almost everything. I wanted only curd rice, pickle, kañji or buttermilk. I drank a bottle of coconut water every morning to help with my morning sickness. I don't know if it was helpful or made my sickness worse. Nellikka (Gooseberry) became my new favourite. We switched to cow's milk from packet milk. We also bought a lot of nuts and dates from a Middle Eastern store - dates from Jordan, pistachios, almonds, cashews, walnuts, macadamia nuts and so much more. But just seeing them sit on the table made me feel like throwing up. I couldn't enjoy any of those.

My doctor had advised me to take rest and be careful for the first three months. So I have been staying at home all the time. No more movie plans or dance plans.

As a dance teacher, the most important time of the year is when we have our Chilañka Pūja or the annual dance program where we have students from different parts of the globe unite together for a week of dancing, learning and celebrations at our academy - Temple Steps. We have exams - both theory and practical and it's a proud feeling seeing each one excel in arts. They also love to play dress-up games. The dance hall will be crowded with pretty girls in colourful practice sarees, full of energy and drenched in sweat. The scent of agarbathis and jasmine flowers fills the place. The sound of bells spread euphony even for the little cats and dogs in our neighbourhood.

But this time, it wasn't the same. We had the event planned for December 11th and I was feeling extremely sick. I hate being irresponsible when it comes to professional commitments and I'm definitely not going to state pregnancy as an excuse to get away. One of the boys was to do a Varṇam (The main item in a Bharatanāṭyam program) - Chalame in Nāṭṭaikuriñji rāga for which I had many jathis (A combination of steps recited using syllables) to learn. I was in complete distress. I couldn't sit up straight for a few hours to learn the jathis or tap them. Everything seemed hard because the nausea was ghastly. But to my surprise, the event and the practice sessions went off remarkably well. My disciple Nakshatra helped me manage a few classes by demonstrating and giving extra practice to others. There were students from Ireland, Dubai, Denmark, Bangalore, Chennai and Kochi and everyone were super supportive. As always we conducted the event with exemplary planning and I felt that my little one was supporting me from the inside. I wore a red silk saree that Nithesh gifted my mom for her birthday. Sivaprasad, the mridañgist said that I have drastically improved in my Naṭṭuvañgam (Tapping and reciting the jathis). I'm grateful to my teachers for all the lessons they have given me. Students were happy and everyone parted by bidding farewell.

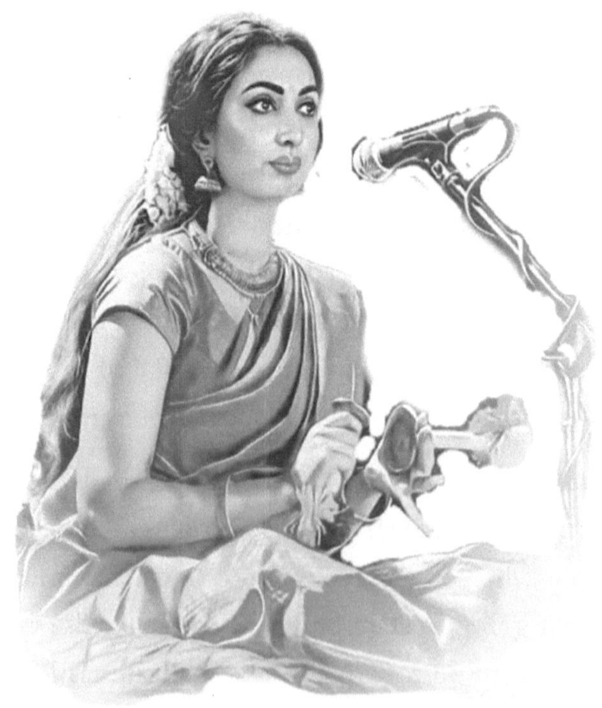

Then came so many days of rest. More nausea, more sleeping and more aversions. I figured out that a lot of times it wasn't vomiting, it was just burping and that was relieving. I vomited twice in that whole trimester and that's it. I made sure to drink milk - at least three glasses. And to my surprise, milk helped with the nausea. How strange! I tried to have boiled eggs every morning. Orange juice became a part of my night routine, and so did pomegranate and buttermilk during the day. Honestly, I did not miss coffee or tea. And Beer? Ew no no no!

Valyamma's natural home remedy

Having a soup with tomato and ginger helps with vomiting during pregnancy. Boil one tomato and a piece of ginger in a pot of water. Let it cool for some time and then blend it with a pinch of salt. Heat the mix once again and add pepper and some butter on top to make it a tasty tangy tomato soup.

THE MILK MAGIC

Milk is a part of many people's diets. With all the lactose intolerance information and vegan diets getting sudden publicity it is natural to wonder if milk is good in pregnancy. And if it is, then, which milk is good during pregnancy?

Milk is good in pregnancy as it is a good source of essential nutrients such as calcium and vitamin D. Milk proteins, especially whey proteins, provide high amounts of essential amino acids and glutamine, both of which help in cell growth and anabolism. However, one should be careful to avoid overconsumption of milk because it may lead to problems like obesity and may have long-term adverse health effects.

BENEFITS OF MILK IN PREGNANCY

Milk increases the calcium intake that is essential for maintaining the bone and teeth density of the mother.

Milk is a good source of minerals such as phosphorus, magnesium, selenium, potassium, and zinc, which are important for the health of both the mother and the growth of the child.

Milk contains water-soluble vitamins like vitamin B1, B2, and B12, and fat-soluble vitamins like vitamin A, D, E, and K, which are essential for the foetus.

Milk is said to promote healthy birth weight in the baby and is also a source of protein, which is important for foetal development.

Milk's high calcium and protein content acts as an antacid, providing relief from heartburn and nausea during pregnancy. A cup of cold milk before bed can help prevent heartburn at night.

It is safe to drink only pasteurised milk during pregnancy. During pasteurisation, milk is heated to a high temperature to kill hazardous microorganisms. However, because raw milk is not sanitised in this manner, it can include dangerous pathogens such as Salmonella and Toxoplasma. One of the most dangerous is Listeria, which can cause listeriosis - a serious infection. Pregnant women are especially vulnerable to Listeria, the top cause of fatal food poisoning. In addition, premature labour, stillbirth, and listeriosis are all potentially fatal for newborns.

According to experts, cow's milk is considered the healthiest kind of milk to drink during pregnancy as it has a great nutritional profile and contains a wide range of vitamins and nutrients like calcium, protein, and vitamin D. While goat's milk contains more calcium, B6, vitamin A, and potassium than cow's milk, it also has more calories and saturated fat than whole cow's milk and contains less B12. Experts also do not recommend buffalo milk during pregnancy because it is high in fat content, and is heavier and harder to digest.

The naturally available sugar in cow's milk is known as lactose. For some women, this may cause bloating or diarrhoea and that is when they are termed lactose intolerant. In such cases, you may try other animal milk options or switch to plant-based milk if you're a vegan by choice.

THE HOLY COW!

In the Hindu culture, the cow occupies a special place. She symbolizes Dharma - the law of righteousness, maternity, wealth and selflessness. A mother can provide milk for the baby only up to three or a maximum of four years after which cow's milk is used as an alternative. That is why the animal is equated to one's mother, hence the expression 'Gau-mātā' (cow mother). In the Hindu tradition, the cow represents both the mother and the earth. Everything produced by the cow is used beneficially in Indian culture. Pañchagavya - the five products of the cow - milk, curd, ghee, urine and dung are purificatory and medicinal. Pañchagavya is used in religious practices, as a medicine and in every aspect of life.

Śiva as Paśupati is the lord of all animals, of which the cow is the foremost. Paśu is cognate with the Latin Pecu, from which are derived words about money, such as pecūnia (Latin) and impecunious (English). Since the Vedic period, the cow has been considered a fortune as it brings wealth into the family. Cattle were essential to the economy. Wealth was estimated by the number of heads of cattle owned either by an individual or the community. Lord Kṛṣṇa is also called Gopāla- a cowherd.

In the Indus Valley civilization, there was very early domestication of cattle, as indicated on the seals, potsherds and terracotta figurines.

There's also a story that says the Greeks named Europe after Europa, once a phoenician maiden desired by Zeus whom Hera turned into a cow and chased westwards.

The Hindus believe in Ahimsa (Non-violence) and regard all animals as sacred. It is not only the four Vedas that condemn the killing of cows. Buddhists and Jains regard cows as sacred animals. The sanctity of the cow was so great that Babur, the first Mughal emperor, in his will to his son Humayun, advised him to respect the cow and avoid cow slaughter. The Mughal king Akbar also chose to ban cow slaughter.

Even though the Constitution of India has banned cow slaughter, very few states actually follow this rule. Cows are brought up in filthy environments and over-milked for their high demand. Male cows are not taken care of while female cows are injected to get pregnant again and again. These places are also breeding grounds for infections.

PLANT-BASED ALTERNATIVES FOR MILK

OAT MILK

Oats are considered essential during pregnancy as they are rich in vitamin B6, calcium and iron. They're also a great source of complex carbohydrates, unsaturated fats and quality protein, containing six of the eight essential amino acids.

SUNFLOWER SEED MILK

They contain high-quality plant protein including all essential amino acids. High levels of unsaturated fatty acids, folic acids and minerals such as calcium and magnesium make them a great choice.

SESAME MILK

Not only does this lovely milk provide you with lots of unsaturated fats, but it's also a great source of vitamins A and B6 (among others). It's also very high in minerals, such as calcium and iron.

ALMOND MILK

Almond is a great source of folic acid, calcium, protein, iron and vitamins A and B6. It's also a great option to avoid gaining too much weight during pregnancy and it protects the baby from developing allergies in the future.

WALNUT MILK

Walnuts, just like the rest of nuts, contain a great amount of polyunsaturated fatty acids which include omega 3 and omega 6. This protects the vascular system. Walnuts are highest in vitamin B6 and vitamin C, both of which are key during pregnancy. Mineral-wise, we see that walnuts are rich in calcium and protein-wise, they're rich in arginine - an essential amino acid.

CASHEW MILK

Cashews are considered as rich food for a reason. Because they are rich in plant protein and unsaturated fats, which support the heart and nervous system during pregnancy. They're also a great source of iron, calcium, vitamin B complex and D.

Mummy and Cheriyammas (Aunts) came to visit me with a lot of gifts during Christmas time. It was the time of cakes. Many knew that I loved red velvet and the fridge was filled with many red velvet cakes and cupcakes with cream cheese frosting. My husband's cousin, Nikitha spent a day with me; Aanu - my best friend - sent cakes, Krishna another close friend from school, visited me a couple of times and some of my students came home in the evenings to talk about nothing and everything till it was dinner time. Many of my friends tried to spend time with me. I looked forward to having visitors at home. Meanwhile, my cousin Ritvik got engaged to a Tamil Brahmin girl - Sriya. I had sister duties on stage and the ceremonies were quite riveting. I wore a yellow silk saree with aqua blue jewellery that I wore for my wedding reception. Two days later, we hosted dinner for them and their parents. Kavya chechi and little Mamatti spent a day with us.

Nithesh used to tell me that when the baby comes, I can drive around with my little one in a Mini Cooper like one of those sassy super cool moms. I thought it was a far-fetched dream. But one fine morning, he told me "Hey Uttu, let's go out and buy a Mini" as simple as going out and buying an ice cream. And just like that we owned our first luxury car.

We got a godmother kind of maid on the day we found out our baby's heartbeat. She was from West Bengal. Sweet girl with a warm heart. In less than a few days, she learned each person's routine and taste. She took care of each one of us, massaged my legs, cooked delicious meals and was such a blessing to our family. She made pazhampori (banana fry) and cheese garlic bread for us in the evenings. Since she was petite, all my pre-pregnancy clothes fit her well. And she was acing all my previous looks. We also got a nice driver from Manipur. Pregnancy and postpartum can be easy when you have so many hands to help. I have had it really easy with having family and house help throughout. I have always loved cooking and driving and I was always on my own. But the person you are during your pregnancy is completely different from the person you were five years ago. So when in need, don't hesitate to ask for help.

I bought a few books so that I could avoid screen time, especially during the night because I have heard that the blue light is unhealthy for the growing foetus and it is important to keep gadgets away at least two hours before bed. The major developments in the womb happen during the night when the mother is asleep. This is the time when the baby is most active. Hence it is important to avoid anything that's harmful to their development right before bed.

But I did not feel like reading. I did not enjoy watching movies, painting or writing. I tried to learn the basics of Mridañgam from YouTube as we had my grandfather's Mridañgam at home which must be at least a hundred years old. I thought I would practice for a few days and then approach a professional to seek guidance but I lost interest within a couple of days. Reciting Viṣṇu and Lalitā Sahasranāmam became a daily evening routine during the time of dusk.

The old saying is that if the first temple you visit after conceiving is that of a Goddess, you are likely to have a girl child and if the presiding deity of the temple is a male God, you might be having a boy. We visited Ponneth Bhagavati temple to take our students before Chilañka Pūja so I think it could be a girl. But Nithesh says that we visited Guruvāyūr after my birthday weekend when we did the Vāhana Pūja for our Innova Crysta. So basically, if we had conceived in Mumbai, Guruvāyūr would be the first temple I visited. That's just a lot of confusion.

WHAT IS AN OLD WIVES' TALE?

The idea of authenticity of an old wives tale is definitely outdated in today's world. But the origins are quite interesting. "Wives" actually refer to women in general as it comes from the English word "wif" and German word "weib" both meaning women. Older women in the family always passed down stories from their experiences - myths, superstitions, and possibilities to the younger generations. Without access to Google at our fingertips, we sometimes gave ourselves into these. Let's take a few old wives' tales and ponder into their scientific truths.

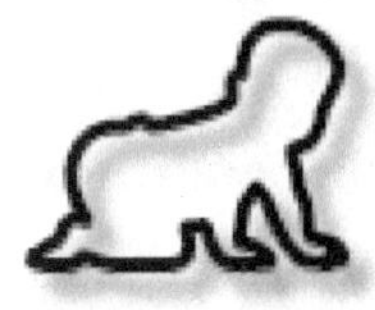

OLD WIVES' TALE - If the expecting mother looks bright and fresh, it could mean she's having a baby girl. But if the expecting mother looks dull and tired, it could mean she's having a baby boy.

Well, it is obvious that the woman's skin will change during her pregnancy due to the changes in her hormones and internal changes in her body. It has nothing to do with the gender of the foetus. Your body may respond differently to the increase or decrease in estrogen or progesterone, iron levels, vitamin levels etc.

SKIN CONDITIONS DURING PREGNANCY

While you have always heard about the pregnancy glow, you may be wondering why you suddenly lost all your charm and charisma. Don't worry, these are a few common skin conditions during pregnancy and the best part is that they will most likely disappear after delivery.

SKIN DARKENING

Melasma or Chloasma - It is common for some women to develop dark patches on their skin during pregnancy. It may appear like a mask around the upper lip, cheeks, neck or forehead. It may appear darker in the areas that are already pigmented like the nipples, genitals etc. These dark patches appear extensively on areas with more friction like underarms or inner thighs. But don't worry, this condition is temporary and could vanish away on its own after the delivery. Melasma may be triggered by hormonal changes that increase the production of melanin in the body. Melanin is the natural source in the body that gives colour to skin and hair. Skin darkening could also be related to the mother's general complexion, stress levels, sun exposure or certain medications.

All changes in skin pigmentation due to melasma usually disappear on their own after delivery, but you can use sun protection with SPF 30 or higher as the UV radiation causes pigmentation to get worse. Nevertheless, it is safe to avoid creams or serums that contain steroids during this period.

ACNE

Acne is common during pregnancy and it may occur severely for those who are prone to acne in general. The increase in hormone levels during this time boosts your skin's production of natural oils. This causes your pores to clog leading to bacterial infections and inflammation.

Acne is the last thing that should bother you during your pregnancy. It is best to avoid any oral medication to treat acne while you're pregnant. Isotretinoin, a drug that is used to treat acne, is said to cause serious birth defects. Antibiotics like tetracycline can inhibit bone growth and discolour the teeth permanently. Most topical medications, acne face washes and creams contain retinoids and they need to be strictly avoided during pregnancy and breastfeeding. Any product containing salicylic acid is also said to harm the developing baby.

Topical treatments containing azelaic acid or erythromycin or over-the-counter products that contain benzoyl peroxide or glycolic acid are considered safe during pregnancy. Only 5% of the medication applied on the skin would be absorbed into the body so it is believed that they may not increase the risk of birth defects.

Muthaśśi's natural home remedy

Pluck a handful of neem leaves and tulsi and crush them into a paste. Add a few drops of squeezed lime or apple cider vinegar to this mixture and apply it on the infected area. Citrus fruits or apple cider contains alpha hydroxy acids. Adding a few drops of honey to this may also help as it works as a natural antiseptic. This clears up the pimples without causing any harm to your baby.

STRETCH MARKS

Most women gain about 10-15 kgs during their pregnancy. When the body grows at a rapid rate within a short span, the middle layer of the skin - the dermis - stretches and tears. This results in the appearance of stretch marks. Applying any natural moisturiser will help reduce the appearance of stretch marks by providing more elasticity to the skin. Stretchy skin may also cause itchiness in the second and third trimesters. Itching may cause the marks to stay on your skin permanently. Apply cocoa butter, bio oil or coconut oil on the stomach, hips and breasts regularly from the second trimester to help the skin stretch. Remember that it is very difficult to get rid of them once they appear. So it is important to take care of them before further damage is done.

But whatever is done to prevent them, it may not be possible to completely get rid of stretch marks. They are called the mask of pregnancy and we may have to accept them with grace.

There might be various skin and hair issues during pregnancy and postpartum. Your body is doing a lot of work creating a tiny human being from scratch. So don't expect sudden results after giving birth but your skin mostly changes back to normal within a couple of months after delivery.

DANDRUFF

Sudden hormonal changes during gestation can send mixed signals to the scalp to increase oil production and generate new skin cells. This excess oil makes way for fungus to grow. When this combines with the older skin cells that are replaced, it leads to hair dandruff. Wash your hair frequently with pregnancy-safe shampoos that contain Ketoconazole - an anti-fungal agent.

Several other conditions may get triggered suddenly during your pregnancy. Spider veins can make you look gruesome but they are harmless and would go away on their own. Some have complained about head lice. This could be due to the oil production in the scalp and also due to the oil head massages many women do during their prenatal period. Some may develop itchy rashes or red bumps on the stomach, thighs, buttocks etc. The skin can get dry or develop a different texture. The texture of hair and nails may also change during pregnancy. All these are bound to occur as the body is preparing for a massive change but don't worry, most of them are reversible.

BEAUTY CARE - WHAT IS SAFE AND UNSAFE?

WAXING AND THREADING

Waxing and threading are generally considered safe during pregnancy but if you have sensitive skin or skin which suddenly started showing changes during pregnancy, waxing could cause more irritation to the already damaged layer of skin. Acne, ingrown hair, redness etc. could be a few results to be expected. Do not wax, shave or thread if you have melasma, varicose veins, rashes, scar tissue or anything unusual.

FACIALS, MANICURES AND PEDICURES

They are safe during pregnancy but be very careful about the hygiene involved in these procedures. UV radiation used for gel polish procedures may harm the skin according to a few studies but there is not much evidence on this topic.

HAIR COLOUR, HAIR SPA, HAIR TREATMENTS

Amonia-free hair colours are safe during pregnancy but strictly refrain from chemical treatments such as hair botox, keratin treatment, smoothening, straightening or rebonding which may require the use of formaldehyde which is a potential carcinogen. Natural hair spas using oil massage or homemade hair packs are safe during pregnancy.

BOTOX, FILLERS, CHEMICAL PEELS

It is best to avoid all such treatments in pregnancy.

LASER HAIR TREATMENTS

There is not enough data to prove that lasers are safe during pregnancy. So it is best to avoid them.

TATTOO

Tattoos are a big no during pregnancy as they increase the chances of infections like HIV, Hepatitis etc. Also, the ink may get into the bloodstream causing harm to the foetus.

WEEKLY DEVELOPMENTS IN THE FIRST TRIMESTER

WEEK 1

The body is preparing for the possibility of a pregnancy. The lining of the uterus is starting to thicken.

WEEK 2

Ovulation happens and the eggs in the fallopian tubes are ready to merge with the sperm. This is when conception happens.

WEEK 3

The new cell that is formed is called zygote which multiplies at a rapid rate as it travels through the fallopian tubes to the uterus becoming a tiny ball called a blastocyst. The blastocyst hatches and implants itself in the anterior or posterior wall of the uterus. The blastocyst contains an embryoblast and a trophoblast.

WEEK 4

Once the cluster has settled into the uterus, it divides into two halves - the placenta and the baby. The baby is now an embryo which is about 0.2mm long. The amniotic sac and the yolk sac are developing at this stage to protect the baby. The heart rate and weight are unknown at this point. The embryo divides into three layers. The inner layer known as endoderm becomes the digestive system, pancreas, thyroid etc. The middle layer known as mesoderm becomes the reproductive organs, bones, kidneys and muscles. The outer layer known as ectoderm becomes the spine, nerves, eyes, teeth, hair etc.

WEEK 5

The tiny embryo is growing at a rapid rate and pregnancy discomforts start for the mother like sore breasts and fatigue. The length of the embryo is now 2mm. Arm and leg buds appear. The placenta and umbilical cord start developing. The placenta is the transfer point between the mother and the baby providing nutrition until delivery.

WEEK 6

The baby's head starts taking shape with the nose, mouth and ears that are beginning to form. The mother may be having morning sickness. The length of the foetus is now 4mm and the heart rate can be seen through an ultrasound.

WEEK 7

The embryo starts forming eyelids and tongue. The uterus has now doubled in size, the heart rate would be between 145-180 bpm and the trunk of the baby would be straightening out more.

WEEK 8

The baby would be moving but you may not feel anything. The length would be 1.3 cm. In rare cases, morning sickness goes beyond typical and into a condition called Hyperemesis Gravidarum. The expecting mother will experience severe vomiting, giddiness and fatigue. Hospitalisation may be required in such rare cases.

WEEK 9

The baby would be the size of a grape and would start looking more human. The head would be bigger than the body. Organs like liver, spleen and gallbladder start developing. The mother may notice her waist broadening, a change in her moods or heartburn.

WEEK 10

The most critical part of development has taken place. The baby's organs are in place and ready to grow. The length would be 3.5 cm weighing about 8 grams. The mother starts to notice a sensitivity towards smell and taste.

WEEK 11

The baby's hands will soon open and close into fists and tiny tooth buds start appearing underneath the gums. Length would be 4.5 cm and weight would be approximately 10 grams. The mother's appearance may be changing and the stomach may start showing for some women. Headache may occur in some women and chromosomal abnormality tests are performed at this period.

WEEK 12

The little toes can curl and the brain is growing at a rapid rate. The baby's internal organs mature and the kidneys are starting to excrete urine. The baby is now weighing about 18 grams with a heart rate between 145-170 bpm and would be 6 cm long. Some women experience dizziness as a symptom of pregnancy.

WEEK 13

The baby now has developed his/her own unique fingerprints and is almost 3 inches long and weighs about 30 grams. Reflex actions like sucking the thumb happen during this stage. Fine hair covers the entire body of the baby to protect it from the amniotic fluid. This is called Lanugo. The baby will be the size of a plum during the end of the first trimester.

NUTRITION DURING THE FIRST TRIMESTER

The simplest mantra for food during pregnancy is to have food that's easy to cook and easy to digest. Always go for what's grown in your locality. From lentils to fruits and veggies, whatever is grown on your land in that particular climate will be healthier. For example, do not go for imported frozen mangos when it's not the season. It will not help in providing the nutritional benefits.

During the first three months, the focus is mainly on retaining the foetus. The diet of the mother has to ensure that the foetus remains stable and there is no bleeding from the vagina. One needs to be careful as bleeding occurring during the initial three months can lead to loss of the foetus.

Iron is a common supplementation women need to take throughout pregnancy. This is because pregnant women need 20-30 mg of iron per day to bear the physiological stresses. Low Hb levels will make it hard for the body to carry oxygen and nutrients which leave you fatigued. This increases the risk of infections and may result in low birth weight for the baby.

Vitamin C helps in better absorption of iron and prevents your chances of catching allergies or flu. Citrus fruits like gooseberry, oranges and lime needed to be added to your diet.

Vitamin B12 also helps in the absorption of iron. Curd or buttermilk not only helps in tackling nausea or vomiting but also helps the gut bacteria.

Nuts, seeds and dry fruits rich in fats and minerals need to be taken during this period. Try to include them in your milkshakes or chew them raw.

Try to avoid coffee, chocolates, green teas, packaged foods, biscuits, breads etc. to keep yourself healthy.

Our ancestors say that cooking food in iron kadais or pans or having food from silver plates also helps in the absorption of iron.

Lean meat like beef, pork and chicken are good sources of protein, iron, choline and other B vitamins. Choline is critical to prevent many gestational issues.

One important ingredient to be added to your diet is asafoetida (Kāyam). It is a common Indian herb that works as an antibiotic and anti-viral. It helps in better digestion and absorption of nutrients. You can use it in curries like sāmbār or rasam, add it to curd rice or drink it in buttermilk. Adding a pinch of it in coconut oil and massaging on your tummy helps in relief from bloating.

Drinking lukewarm water boiled with cumin (jīrakam) also helps with gas. Cumin can be had in various forms as it's an important ingredient in North Indian recipes.

Rāgī or millet is a gluten-free food rich in amino acids, calcium, iron and fibre. It regulates our appetite and in the long term helps in lactation too. You can have it as a malt with milk, make laddoos, dosas or rotis out of it as per your choice.

Beetroot and green apple are great sources of folic acid. Folate supports healthy pregnancy. It is said that beetroot leaves also help in preventing varicose veins which is a common concern during pregnancy.

Some say you need to eat for two which is not necessary. You need to eat the right kind of food to get the right kind of nutrition needed for your body. Try to divide your meals into smaller portions. Like if you're having three main meals, divide them into six half-quantity meals. This will keep the acidity down and keep you feeling full throughout. Keep a snack ready to munch in the middle of the night too as taking an eight-hour gap at night may worsen the nausea in the morning. Maybe that's the reason it is called morning sickness!

ABORTION

A spontaneous loss of pregnancy before the first 20 weeks starting from the first week of your last period is known as an abortion or a miscarriage. It has been found that 10 to 15% of clinically diagnosed pregnancies may result in a miscarriage. Their causes vary according to several conditions, especially the trimesters.

Here are a few common causes for first-trimester abortions:

- The most common cause for malformations or miscarriage is Chromosomal/Congenital abnormality in the foetus. This is completely not in your hands and therefore it is tested in the first trimester itself to identify genetic problems. This test is known as Karyotyping.
- Medical experts say that an increase in maternal age may lead to miscarriages.
- Those who are suffering from chronic medical conditions like hypertension, diabetes, kidney diseases, autoimmune diseases etc. and those who suffer from hormonal disorders like hyperthyroidism or hypothyroidism, PCOD, increase in prolactin levels etc. may have an increased chance for abortions.

- Smoking, drugs and alcohol definitely increase the chances for abortions.
- Being underweight or overweight could affect your pregnancy.
- Exposure to environmental toxins like lead and mercury may also lead to miscarriages.
- Antiphospholipid Syndrome or Acquired Thrombophilia is a condition where the blood vessels thicken and clots are formed on the blood vessels towards the uterus which block the passage resulting in the death of the foetus.

Research shows that miscarriages are more common in the first trimester than in the second trimester. If miscarriages occur more than three consecutive times, it is known as Recurrent Pregnancy Loss or RPL.

Here are a few common causes for second-trimester abortions:

- Infections of the genital tract or the pelvis could be one of the reasons for an abortion.
- High-grade fever at any time of the pregnancy can end in miscarriages.
- Cervical incompetence is a condition where the cervix is weak and starts dilating before the pregnancy completes its term. In such cases, the doctor stitches the cervix until the baby is full term.
- Uterine fibroids, uterine abnormalities, growths or polyps in the uterus etc. can also increase the risks.

If the baby dies after 20 weeks of pregnancy, it is called a foetal demise or stillbirth. This is extremely rare but there is still a possibility. For abortions beyond this stage, the woman is most commonly made to go through the procedures of normal labour. Rest and recovery are very crucial after this procedure.

Studies suggest that 90% of women have normal pregnancies after a miscarriage and only 1% of women go through recurrent miscarriages.

There are treatments available for anything and everything with the advancement of medical studies. In case of recurrent miscarriages, check with your doctor for further evaluation. Hysteroscopy is a procedure done by inserting an endoscope internally to examine the uterine cavities. 3-D scans are also available at hospitals for evaluation. Get enough care for yourself throughout your pregnancy and keep your doctor informed about any difficulty you are facing.

When an abortion occurs, it can be extremely painful mentally and sometimes physically to the woman. This can be an emotionally devastating phase for the mother as well as the entire family. But it is better to understand it from such a perspective that nature is protecting you from giving birth to an abnormal baby by terminating the pregnancy naturally. The woman now needs more support from her loved ones and when she is mentally stable and physically back to normal, in optimum health, she can check with her doctor and plan for a pregnancy once again.

THE SECOND TRIMESTER

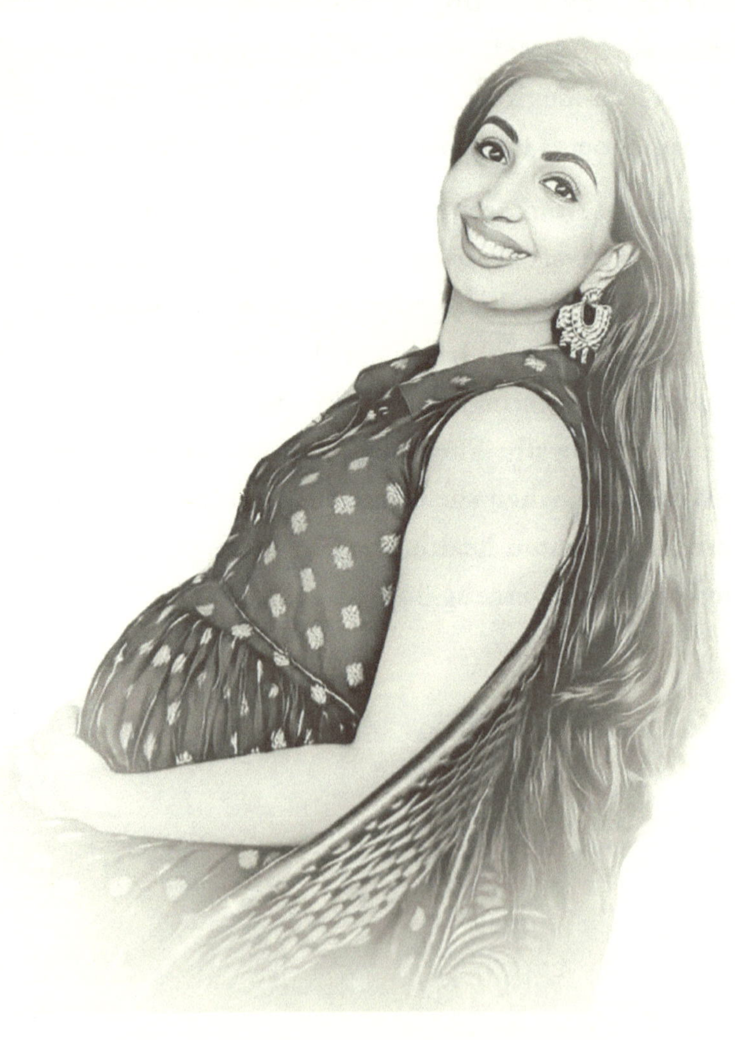

Time for bigger clothes and bigger lingerie! I was a universal XS - Extra Small. And now I don't even know what fits me. Every day things kept getting tighter for me. This was getting scary. Am I supposed to keep buying new clothes every month from now? Am I ever going to get back to an XS?

By around 16 weeks, I started feeling a lot more better. I started going for evening walks in our beautiful colony - Neptune Country. I always feel I live in a breathtakingly picturesque society. I can't get over the beauty of this place. The lush green verdancy, the serene backwaters covering this area, the artistic monuments created by Sri. Kaladharan - Kilithara and Kalithara, the open space and the gardens of each villa filled with a myriad of different flowers. Every villa is divided by traditional white picket fencing which is the trademark of this property. We can often see birds of different varieties - The green parrots that are a rare visual treat, the loud bulbul with its black and red vivid colours, the famous mynah and many others. We had a swimming pool since 2005 or so, a time when pools/gyms were not a common part of communities, at least in Kochi. I loved early morning swims with my dad or in the nights with my mom. The blue tiles of the open-air pool blazed the luminescence from the moon and stars. Sometimes I'd take Momo, our cocker spaniel, along and tie her close by like she was there to guard me when I went swimming alone. If you're someone who grew up with dogs, you'd be a natural mom. Dog moms have a natural instinct to nurture, love, care and protect unconditionally.

Kalithara is an open stage in Neptune. I think as a dancer, I am extremely blessed to have a stage exclusively for myself. Before a main event I'd spend days rehearsing in my dance studio and then like a final rehearsal, we'd sometimes invite friends and family to watch my mini performance at Kalithara. The aunts of Neptune always encouraged my ventures. So did the birds and trees in this neighbourhood that sing and dance along with me.

EXERCISE

"Your body will be around a lot longer than that expensive handbag. Invest in yourself."

In earlier times, women were not exposed to the comfort of Western toilets or attached bathrooms. They had to walk a couple of miles to take a bath in the pond or river nearby. Even a few years later, most houses had their bathrooms/toilets outside the main compound. Western commodes became common in India probably after the 1980s. Till then squatting a couple of times a day was a must at least to pee and poop. The faddish dining tables too became common in our households around the 1960s. So every meal had to be taken by sitting on the floor. These simple lifestyle changes over the decades have deteriorated our physical health and fitness. Pregnant women were not over-pampered like how it is done today.

Exercise improves a person's general health and well-being and when it is done appropriately, it can be aimed at promoting a normal and smooth delivery. Nonetheless, it totally depends on your medical conditions. Each body is different. So always get confirmation from your obstetrician before attempting any physical activity.

There are several benefits of exercising during pregnancy. Not only that exercise keeps your energy levels better, they produce hormones called endorphins that enhance your mood and improve sleep quality. Exercise helps with swelling, pelvic pain and backaches if done in the right manner. If it worsens any of these conditions, stop immediately and continue only with the help of a professional. Any activity should not exceed 30 minutes and always listen to your body. If you experience excessive panting, pain, giddiness etc., you need to stop immediately. Exercise reduces the risk of complications like gestational diabetes, preeclampsia and chances of cesarean deliveries. Exercise increases blood flow to the placenta which improves the baby's health as well. Above all, exercise keeps you fit and prepares you for labour and delivery.

While you're pregnant, make sure not to overdo any exercise. Avoid activities that involve jumping or skipping or anything where falling is more likely because your weight is changing at a rapid rate, your centre of gravity is shifting too soon and you may lose balance if you don't take enough care. Drink plenty of water to stay hydrated.

Here are a few exercises that you can include during your pregnancy:

- Walking is one of the safest forms of exercise you can do unless you have been advised bed rest by your doctor.
- Squats improve the strength of your thigh muscles and give you a better birthing position.
- Kegels aids in strengthening the pelvic floor muscles.
- Pelvic tilts strengthen abdominal muscles and help alleviate back pain during pregnancy.

- **Butterflys help as hip openers that promote better positioning of the baby.**
- **Cat and cow poses assist in relieving trapped gas in the intestines.**
- **Duck walking improves flexibility and promotes normal delivery.**

A woman's body goes through a massive transformation during pregnancy and remember that it is not easy to grow a human being inside. Therefore, it is advisable to work with someone who is certified in pre and postnatal exercise training. An expert can provide you with personalised guidelines based on your health and specific pregnancy needs.

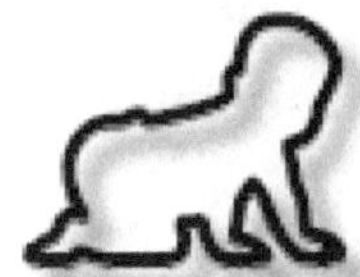

OLD WIVES' TALE - If you are carrying high, you are most likely to have a baby boy and if you are carrying low, you are likely to have a girl.

The shape of your tummy doesn't have anything to do with your pregnancy, the gender of the foetus or the baby's weight. Sometimes a huge tummy could also deliver an underweight baby and the size would just be more of the amniotic fluid. Sometimes a small tummy can give birth to a healthy and well-nourished baby. The shape of your tummy could depend on various factors like your hereditary body shape, your BMI, muscle strength and weight distribution in your body.

PREGNANCY RHINITIS

Sometimes pregnancy can make way for aggravation in allergies for those who are already prone to sinusitis. This condition is known as pregnancy rhinitis. When the blood flow to the nasal passages increases, the nasal veins may get enlarged. When there is water retention in the body, the mucous membranes in your nasal passage may proliferate causing inflammation. This causes congestion in the nasal passage resulting in pregnancy rhinitis.

It could appear anytime during your gestational period in the form of itchy eyes, running nose, sneezing etc. Having extra fluid in the body, high levels of estrogen or the pregnancy hormone called HCG could be the causes of pregnancy rhinitis. Since popping in cetirizine or other flu tablets frequently is not a healthy option during this time, though it is considered safe, it will be good to supplement yourself with vitamin C-rich food or tablets.

Ammuma's natural home remedies -

Saline spray -

You can use saline water as a nasal spray. This would help with better breathing through the nose.

Lime -

Drinking a glass of hot water mixed with a freshly squeezed lemon and a pinch of salt helps as a quick remedy when your allergies start to catch up. Remember to have this immediately after your first sneeze.

Chukku Kāpi -

Add Thulasi, pepper powder, crushed ginger, panikūrka and some crushed jaggery to water and boil the mixture. Let it boil for a few minutes to become a concentrated potion. Drink this hot a few times a day and it should give a lot of relief. Panikūrka is a natural herb that cures fever, painful sinus and urinary infections. Its English name is Plectranthus Amboinicus. Bathing babies and children in water boiled with panikūrka also helps in curing colds, flu or fever in them.

Nellikka (Gooseberry)

Gooseberry works as the best natural substitute for vitamin C. Have it raw or soaked in salt water.

Chechiyamma's home remedy

Roll some turmeric, rāsnādi powder and ghee like a cigar pipe in a piece of thin soft cloth. Burn it and inhale its smoke. Its strong smell will cause a burning sensation in your nose and head but cures cold before you even know it.

OBSTRUCTIVE SLEEP APNEA

Sleep can be elusive during pregnancy and many women may be struggling with sleep. Congestion in the nasal passage may also cause severe snoring in pregnant women. Snoring may lead to disturbed sleep resulting in a condition called obstructive sleep apnea. OSA is caused when the throat muscles relax and narrow your airway. This puts pressure on the air passage. When you can't get enough air, the oxygen in the blood level decreases. The brain senses that you can't breathe and briefly wakes you up to reopen the airway. This is so ephemeral that you might not even remember. This pattern repeats several times every hour throughout the night. While some show symptoms like snoring, some may simply experience fatigue, headache, insomnia, anxiety or depression. This is due to the body not being able to meet its sleep requirements.

Sudden weight gain or water retention in the body may be the causes of sleep apnea during pregnancy and these are not in our control. Doing mild exercises may help with better sleep during this time. It is important to keep your head elevated during sleep so the air passage may not be restricted much. In worst cases,

a CPAP (Continuous positive airway pressure) machine is effective before, during and after pregnancy.

While OSA is not a life-threatening illness, it is not to be taken for granted. OSA during pregnancy can lead to long-term health complications so make sure to shed the pregnancy weight soon after delivery to prevent further complications.

We had Christmas and Thiruvāthira celebrations in Neptune during December and January. The aunties in our colony are all extremely cheerful and enthusiastic. All festivals throughout the year are celebrated here. My mom is usually the one in charge of everything. I don't know where she gets the energy from to teach everyone, coordinate and conduct the events.

End of January I had to make my presence as chief guest for a couple of events. One for a school in Kochi where I even shared the stage with the chief justice of Kerala high court. It felt good to be a speaker on stage after a long time.

I wasn't a smart child. The biggest fear in my life was to hear my own voice come out of my mouth in front of an audience! Talking was always a difficult task, always! I could dance, I could paint, I could write but I could never talk on stage. I used to bunk on days when we were asked to conduct seminars/ give a speech/ lecture demonstrations etc. in school and college. Bringing words out of my mouth was the most challenging thing I ever had to do. But conquering our fears is what makes us feel truly successful, right? When my first film was geared for its release, I was suddenly pushed in front of a hundred cameras to speak up. That was the first time. Little did I know that emceeing was something I'd have to take up later. I think life forces you to take up jobs that you're terrible at to teach you that you can't run away. And the only choice you have is to get better at it. Emceeing, teaching, demonstrating and singing; fifty percent of my work is done by bringing words out of my mouth. And guess what, it isn't all that difficult! I realised that everything is possible if you try.

I was also fortunate to light the inaugural main lamp for the Poñgāla (a temple ritual where women boil rice in a pot as a symbol of prosperity) at Chettikulañgara Bhagavati temple along with Nithesh. Thousands of pots along the way were lit from the main lamp and we consider it an enormous blessing to have had this opportunity during my fourth month of pregnancy.

Students of Temple Steps and I performed at a Murugan temple in Aluva on February 2nd. I had committed myself to this program before I got pregnant and though my students were performing the main parts, I had to make them feel my presence on stage. My favourite student Nitya, was supposed to compensate on my behalf. To everyone's surprise, she didn't turn up for the event. She said she had another program but did not even come to take the blessings, show her item or ask for feedback. I won't deny the fact that it hurt. However, our students performed well. I did a Padam - Sri Rāma Chandra which I choreographed for Nitya's Arañgetram.

Nitya's family owned a small grocery store located on the corner of our street. I'd sometimes buy sipup for Rs. 1/- when I walked back from school, decades ago. I always looked at the cute little toddler who'd be seated on the tabletop. I'd wave at her and she'd say "Tata". That's my first memory of her.

One day, while Amma and I were renovating our terrace into a dance space, soon after I moved back home from Mumbai, Nitya's father asked us what would be the fee structure for the new dance class in town. We were sure they won't be able to afford that kind of an expensive fee so we told him not to worry about it.

She was a beautiful girl, fair-skinned and petite with an innate talent for dance. Her brown curls and brown eyes made her look like she belonged to a different ethnicity. As months passed by, I perfected her technique and style. She became noticeably one of the best performers in our class. Little children looked up to her with fascination in their eyes. Our classes flourished within a year and we had our first annual celebration. Nitya was applauded immensely by the audience for her outstanding performance and she was awarded the best student of the year.

I personally ran the errands of getting copies of her certificates, filling her admission forms and paying to enrol her for a diploma in Bharatanāṭyam. After being rejected twice, she got selected for a graduate course at a prestigious dance college. I was proud of the way she started understanding dance. Dance is not just the tapping to the rhythm and music, it is the poetry of the body.

Despite having nothing in common, I always enjoyed my conversations with Nitya. I loved her outlook towards everything. Greed was not something she'd ever feel. I took her to seven-star hotels, gave her many of my favourite luxe clothes, and made her perform in several TV shows and yet I never saw her eyes sparkle. I thought that was her virtue.

Nitya's big debut was a special day for all of us; it was the first Arañgetram from Temple Steps. We spent days and nights rehearsing together. I'd choreograph a jathi, then make changes, then come up with a new idea and the process went on and on. Most days we'd feed her and make her sleep here because more than her I wanted to make sure she's rested well. I would force her to drink protein shake before she left and so she would run through the backyard before she heard the sound of the blender.

My mother and I hopped from shop to shop in Chennai finding the perfect costume for her Arañgetram. We decided on a bottle green silk saree that would suit her the best. After a few days, I gave her one of my favourite ink blue and gold costume too so that she could have a dress change in the latter half of the recital. We booked one of the best venues in Kochi, picked the best musicians, and planned a grand event. Of course, the budget was beyond what any of us could imagine. But I didn't think twice because she had already become like the sister I never had. That day was a dream come true for all of us. The lighting looked surreal and Murugan's makeup made her look gorgeous. Prashob gave her the original temple jewellery. We had a famous dancer come as the chief guest for the event and her wise words conveyed that the biggest blessing for a student is the right Guru and for a Guru, the right student. I was so proud of her like I could see nothing in her other than a reflection of myself.

But people aren't always as grateful as you expect them to be. I learnt it the hard way that no one stays after they are done. Like how birds fly out of the nest, they aren't yours forever.

Nitya never came to me for classes, she never paid me the costs I had to bear, and she never helped me during my pregnancy to manage my classes. All I heard her tell others was "Oh, no one will stay there forever."

We did not have any paperwork done with conditions but I thought she would be around like family or help me when I was in need. Isn't it a human tendency to have expectations from your loved ones? Parents give their everything to their children and expect them to do the same when they are old and sick. But are people always able to return that favour?

There's a story about spiders. Once the spiders mate, the female spider will eat its partner and when the spider produces offspring, they feed on and consume the mother. This behaviour is known as Matriphagy and is common among many species. The spider represents the importance of perseverance and the essence of existence signifying that everything that is produced by Brahmaṇ ends in Brahmaṇ.

You can teach everything but you can't teach gratitude. I couldn't stop thinking about her while I performed the Padam - It's through the eyes of Lord Rāma's mother. A mother's yearning to meet her beloved son. Sometimes I feel everything happens for a reason. Maybe Nitya had to be ungrateful as a way for the universe to teach me that I shouldn't be expecting anything from my unborn child. Thank you Nitya for teaching me that "Vālsalyam" could hurt. My love for you was endless and unconditional like a sister, a daughter I never had. I only wanted to see you grow and shine. But you never understood how much you meant to me.

Well, thanks to her we started a scholarship program at Temple Steps - without any personal or emotional favouritism, we simply teach the art for free to truly deserving underprivileged students. Charity should not be done with attachments because attachments lead us to expectations. And people can never live up to anyone's expectations.

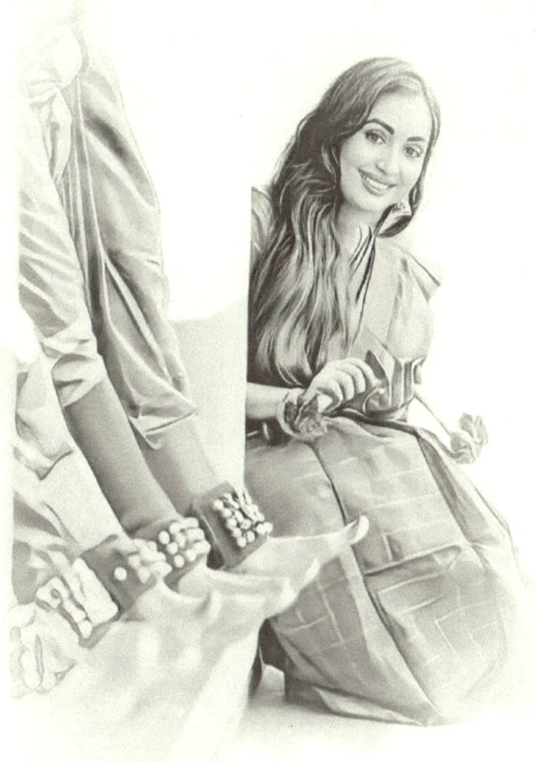

Before one becomes a teacher, she becomes a mother. How much ever we try to draw professional boundaries, we end up loving our students like our own. Are we as dance teachers possessive of our students' art? Do we sometimes feel "Wow I created that" or "That's mine"? That's why we often feel bad when they give up on dancing or when their priorities change and dance becomes of less importance. We feel we invested more time in moulding them than their own personal interest and passion. But what are we possessing? The art or the artist? I don't think any of my teachers ever possessed me, nobody went out of the way to make me better. Of course, my mother did so and continues to do so. As a wise teacher, one needs to act like a wise parent too. Our duty here is to only teach, provide and guide them. As we watched them grow, we watched their art grow too. But reality hits that nothing and no one belongs to us. We are only tools through which the art was passed on. It is neither mine nor yours. The sooner we realise that, the better we can be. We can stay away from personal favouritism and possession. Our duty was only to nurture them. When they grow wings, they will all fly away and we should be happy to see them fly away. Like a proud mother bird, I'll watch my baby birds fly away. There's a lot of sky out there for each one of them...

MOOD SWINGS

"If you want the rainbow, you gotta put up with the rain."

- Dolly Parton

Pregnancy is a time when your body goes through a roller coaster of emotions. You might be oscillating between pure joy and utter despair within a fraction of seconds and you won't be able to figure out why. It's a wild ride full of happy highs and lugubrious lows. Well, not every expecting woman will experience these rapid ups and downs but the good news is that these are all temporary and completely normal.

It is natural to feel worried and stressed at several stages during your pregnancy. However, high levels of stress and anxiety during pregnancy can increase the risk of miscarriage, preterm delivery, and a baby born with less weight. Maternal anxiety early in pregnancy can affect the child's development at a later stage resulting in conditions like Attention Deficit Hyperactivity Disorder (ADHD), Anxiety, Cerebral Palsy etc. In order to avoid all such complications, it is important to take enough care of your mental health during your prenatal period.

HORMONES

The sudden shift in hormone levels could play a major role in contributing to mood swings. During the early stages of gestation, there will be a quick flood of estrogen and progesterone. This could take a toll on one's mental health.

Estrogen works throughout your entire body and is active in the region of the brain that is responsible for your mood. This hormone is associated with anxiety, irritability and depression. Whereas, Progesterone is a hormone that helps to loosen the muscles and joints. It also prevents early contractions. That's why it is sometimes prescribed by doctors to protect the foetus during the early stages of pregnancy. Consequently, progesterone can cause fatigue, nausea, and even uncontrollable crying. Therefore a sudden increase of estrogen and progesterone could cause your mental state to be unstable.

FATIGUE AND SLEEP DEPRIVATION

When your body is tired, you definitely can't be in the best of your moods. The first-trimester fatigue is real and "tired" is just an understatement. No matter how much you sleep or rest, you feel it isn't enough. Sleeping in the third trimester could be another challenge. With all the changes in your body and the heaviness of the growing belly, every position could be uncomfortable. That's why they say the second trimester is more like the honeymoon phase of pregnancy.

MORNING SICKNESS

Morning sickness doesn't cause just physical discomfort, it can be mentally exhausting too. Not knowing when to rush to the toilet or throw up could be irritating. Nausea also doesn't let you enjoy your favourite meal or snack and that is definitely not one of the best feelings at all.

PHYSICAL CHANGES

Your changing body can make you feel extremely happy or exasperatingly sad. It is incredible to feel a tiny human grow inside you but watching your body become unrecognisable can come with its own set of complicated feelings. Your body is creating a wonder. Hang in there and embrace the change.

ANXIETY AND STRESS

There are a million reasons for you to be worried in general. Stress about becoming a parent, life adjustments, finances, labour pain, complications during labour, recovery and postpartum etc. There are endless complications to fret about and it could be unnerving for moms-to-be. If you have had miscarriages in the past, it could be more taxing. Other non-pregnancy-related causes for your anxiety can add fuel to your already unstable mind.

Mood swings vary from person to person and each woman has their own unique feelings. A study from 2015 found that women who report premenstrual mood swings tend to experience them more during their pregnancy. Many women experience excitement and tension all at once and it's not surprising. You may get angry over the pettiest of problems or laugh uncontrollably over something silly. You may cry over things that don't matter or get overwhelmed with the changes coming your way. While there is so much awareness on postpartum depression, we fail to address depression during pregnancy. So if you feel perpetually dismayed, talk to your doctor.

Here are a few things you can do to cope with mood swings:

EAT WELL

If you've ever gotten "hangry," you should know that hunger can lead to an undesirable outburst. You may not understand that you are simply "Hangry" most of the time. Quell your appetite with healthy and nutritious meals, and fuel your body and mind with tasty snacks. This can help you calm your anger. Good food can keep you happy and collected.

GET EXERCISE

Exercise releases endorphins which act as a great stress reliever and mood booster. Mild exercises like walking or swimming could help with better digestion and better sleep. Moreover, the fresh air will refresh and invigorate you. Keep your activity limited between 15-30 minutes and stop if you feel breathless and tired. Listen to your body and act accordingly. However, consult your doctor before you begin any rigorous activity.

YOGA

Yoga and meditation are also immensely helpful to keep you well mentally and physically. If you're not sure where to start there are many tutorial videos online. You can learn to stretch and breathe just to keep yourself calm. But before trying any intense movement, get the help of a professional teacher.

PRIORITISE SLEEP

It's so important to get quality sleep when you are expecting. Maintain a sleep schedule and make it a priority. Your body is creating a human being and it requires a lot of rest. Engage in breathing exercises that help you sleep better and make yourself comfortable with a warm shower before bed. Sleep using a pregnancy pillow. Drink a glass of milk before bed so it helps you fall asleep faster. Also, note that the major developments of the baby in the womb happen while you are sleeping, so make sure you avoid screen time two hours before bed. Therefore no watching movies, playing games or scrolling through social media while hitting the bed.

TALK TO YOUR LOVED ONES

A lot of your mood swings can be managed with helping partners, friends and family. Having people around who understand you and support you for your big change, will make a big difference in your overall well-being. So don't hesitate to seek help or talk to your loved ones when you feel low.

EMBRACE THIS PHASE

Pregnancy is tough. It is okay to feel a sudden load of emotions. Understand that it is your hormones making you feel melodramatic and reward yourself for the big job you are doing. Embrace this phase and let yourself be. It's okay to vent so be kind to yourself and know that these temper tidal waves are temporary.

TALK TO A THERAPIST

If you feel like your emotions are really difficult to manage, you should seek help from a professional. Talk to your obstetrician or a psychologist. Prenatal depression and anxiety are common, and it's nothing to feel ashamed about. Reclaim your mental health with the help of a professional to have a healthy baby.

Mood swings belong to one of the most common, less talked about pregnancy symptoms. Know that these big feelings are all a

part of the journey and they're getting you ready to experience the most overwhelming emotion of them all - unconditional love for your tiny sapling.

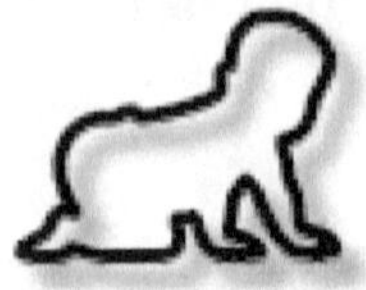

OLD WIVES' TALE - If the pregnant woman is experiencing a lot of morning sickness and vomiting, she's likely to have a girl and if the morning sickness is mild and manageable, she's likely to have a boy.

Sickness of any kind has nothing to do with the baby's gender. Medical experts haven't been able to pinpoint the exact cause of morning sickness but many professionals link it to higher levels of the pregnancy hormone, HCG (Human Chorionic Gonadotropin) and estrogen.

Amma had a serious surgery on February 28th. She had been getting frequent migraines and was always suffering from vertigo. I was getting worried. We consulted various doctors for her sleep apnea and breathing issues. But nothing worked. Dr. Vinu Māma (My uncle) suggested she consult Dr. Radhakrishnan at Medical Trust Hospital. After a head MRI they found a tumour in her pituitary gland. She was suffering from Acromegaly - a condition which causes the body parts to grow large. Her hormones have been fluctuating and that's why she was constantly gaining weight. The tumour which is already big might damage her vision as it would obstruct the optic nerve if it grows further. Hence surgery was the only option - Brain surgery!

We decided to do it in Aster Medcity. Nithesh met Farhaan, the operations head and fixed a consultation with Dr. Dilip Panicker, one of the most credible Neurosurgeons in India. Those weren't happy days. All the brain tumours they showed us through films made us feel extremely apprehensive about this situation.

We left home around 4 PM before Rāhu Kālam and spent some time in Grand Hyatt to sip some coffee before we admitted Amma at Aster. What an irony! A five-star coffee before brain surgery!

On the surgery day, I went to the temple, came back home and started praying until the surgery was done. Viṣṇu and Lalitā Sahasranāmam back to back. During her surgery time, Momo, our cocker spaniel, started howling ghastly which she had done only during Ammuma's passing away. It ran a chill through my spine and I can't explain how petrified I was, being all alone at home. I immediately took Momo inside and put her to sleep and continued praying hard. I was munching on some cheese balls and soda because the little one inside still made me hungry every hour. I knew it was an unhealthy snack, but I wasn't in a sane mindset to care. By lunchtime, Acha called and said that everything went well and she has been brought into the ICU. God, that was a relief! But that night was macabre for her. She couldn't breathe as her nose was packed and there was a huge catheter all the way from her nose to throat. Acha sat beside her in the ICU for hours. Nithesh was also at the hospital. He came back pretty late and I was really upset knowing her condition. She kept on murmuring in her sleep "Pansu varanda… Pansu enne kānanda" and I couldn't stop myself from crying all night.

It was on this day that I had a moment of epiphany - we had never spent a day without speaking to each other. Even if we were travelling in two ends of the globe, even if we fought, even on the busiest of days, we have managed to connect. I know I was overthinking, but that slightest fear of "*what if I don't get to speak to her again?*" made me awfully distressed.

The next day I met my jaunty Amma in the room. Never have I ever seen her so dreary and vulnerable. She was trying to complain to me showing me all the cuts and bandages like how a little child would tell her mom. I have always been her mom more than she was mine. I couldn't stop myself from crying. She kept licking butter to moisturise her extremely dry mouth; she still couldn't swallow anything. That night was also frightful. Removing that massive trumpet kind of tube from her nose without any anaesthetic was excruciatingly painful for her. And by then she was at her weakest. But that put an end to everything. She could now breathe better and swallow thick liquids. I finally slept peacefully but cried saying sorry to my baby for not being able to put her/him as my first priority.

It is so true that when a child is born, a mother is born too. You suddenly start seeing your mother as a mother. Your childhood pictures are not just your pictures anymore. Instead, you see the woman behind those frames who took an effort to dress you up, make you smile and frame those images in between her sleep-deprived days. Amma keeps a little diary where she has written about all my firsts. The surprising fact is that she still continues to fill that book. She remembers my performance dates or accolades more than I myself would. A mother is a mother forever, however grown her child is.

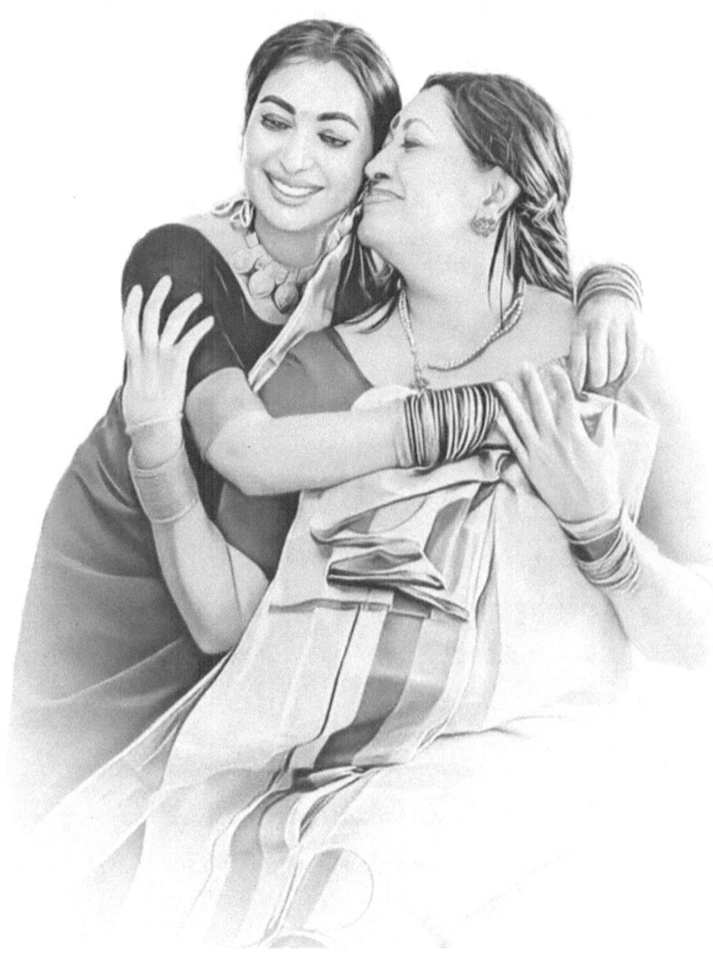

I couldn't help but wonder, how many of us are lucky enough to carry our first friendships forward forever? Even as we grow, even as we mature, even as our attitudes, interests and priorities change.

But some bonds grow stronger with time. Amma was my first friend who taught me to laugh, who taught me to speak, who taught me to walk… I grew up without siblings and she was my world until I went to school. She was still my best friend throughout my teenage and adulthood. She was so amazing in understanding all my teen issues and keeping all my secrets. When I received my first love letter, when a boy proposed to me for the first time, when I went on my first date… She was cooler than friends my age. She became my travel buddy later and my forever best friend. The fun nights in Thailand, the trekking in Manali, and the sightseeing in Nepal, we have had enough and more fun dance travels together. As fun as the trips sound, she was always my best cheerleader and my worst critic. My first dance Guru and mentor in everything I have ever done. She's more than just a best friend but I call her mom.

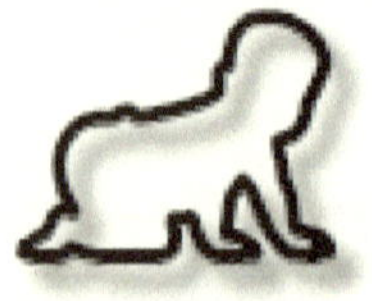

OLD WIVES' TALE - If you're happy and jovial during the period of your pregnancy, it could mean that you're having a boy and if you're prone to mood swings that lead you to be cranky and upset about little things, you could be having a girl.

Pregnancy and mood swings are like a couple. Irrespective of what gender you have conceived, your hormones would bring changes to the way you feel about things around you. Therefore it has nothing to do with your baby's gender.

WATER

Sometimes you will end up paying a price if you take the simplest and most important things for granted. Hydrating yourself frequently is essential, especially during pregnancy. This is a time when blood volume increases by 45%. Symptoms of mild dehydration include headaches, fatigue, bad mood and in worst cases, reduced memory. 8-12 glasses of water per day is required for a pregnant body. If your body fails to meet its water requirements it can result in constipation or urinary tract infections. Keep a personal reusable bottle to measure your water intake to avoid complications. Using a copper bottle is healthier as your body will also receive the absorbed metal. You may use glass or steel bottles too as a sustainable choice and try to refrain from plastic.

YONIJA - AYONIJA

Yonija is a normal human being who is born from the uterus of a woman. But in the Purāṇas, we come across the concept of Ayonija - someone who is not born from the womb, and consequently, can bypass or rise above the cycle of birth and death. He who is born out of self is Swayambhu. Śiva is Swayambhu.

According to Buddhist and Hindu mythology, birth from the female body brings one into the circle of life and death, or samsāra. So, the one who is born out of a woman's womb, or Yonija, experiences birth as well as death. Lord Rām who lived in Tretāyuga was born from the womb of Kauśalya and lord Kṛṣṇa who lived in Dvāparayuga was born from the womb of Devaki. Hence, both of them experienced death.

The story of Gaṇeṣa is an interesting case. Gaṇeṣa was not born from a mother's womb, he was created. One day when Pārvati Devi was preparing for her bath, she wondered if there was anyone to guard her. She suddenly had an idea and created a mould of a little boy from the turmeric and sandalwood paste she was applying on her body. She gave the cute little boy a life and asked him to guard her while she took her bath. When lord Śiva appeared, he was denied entry by the little one. This led to a fight between them resulting in the death of the little boy. Pārvati is now furious with Śiva for chopping off her son's head. Śiva immediately replaces the head with the life of a dying elephant and the new form that's brought to life is a little God with elephant face and human body - Gaṇeṣa!

Similarly, Śiva's other son Kārtikeya was also not born from a mother's body. Śiva's seed first falls in fire, then in wind, and finally, in the river - Gañga, setting the riverbank reeds aflame. From the ashes emerges Kārtikeya, as the six-headed warlord.

Another son of Śiva was born when Śiva merges with Viṣṇu who came in the form of Mohini to become Harihara. Two male Gods thus come together and a child is created. This child is Ayappa.

Other such characters in mythology who are not womb-born are also well-known. There is the famous story of Mandhata - A king of the Ikṣavaku dynasty (Solar). A king called Yuvanaṣwa accidentally drinks a magic potion which was meant to make women pregnant and, in doing so, becomes pregnant himself. The sages and servants of the kingdom helped the king to give birth. The king's left abdomen was slit open and the child, Mandhata, was born. Mandhata, thus, becomes a special king, having been born in a special way and it is believed that he was very powerful and could conquer the world in a single day.

In later Buddhist stories, there are suggestions that Buddha was not born in the normal way. He was conceived by his mother Māya when she dreamt that a white elephant entered her right side. Buddha was born from the side of his mother, not through the vaginal canal. He was strong enough to walk seven steps as soon as he was born. But Buddha's life also took a fatal turn.

Christianity proclaims how Jesus was conceived immaculately, without sex, to the Virgin Mary and Joseph. He was believed as the saviour and Messiah of the world. But even Jesus Christ had to succumb to death, though he was raised from the dead on the third day after his crucifixion. Thus, the woman's body came to be associated with death and the cycle of rebirth.

In Tantra parampara, it is said that the world began with Devi who was called Prakrti. She is also called Trayamba because she gave birth to three eggs from which were born Brahma, Viṣṇu and Maheśvara. In Vaiṣṇava parampara and Śiva parampara, God is Swayambhu.

Yamini chechi, one of Amma's first students, came to stay with us to take care of mom post-surgery. How easy and fast is the recovery now? The medical world has advanced to great heights. Since Amma's surgery was through a nasal invasive procedure, there are no marks or scars on her head or face. She's lost weight and looks ten years younger now.

Due to all the strain and improper supplementation, I started getting severe stomach pain. When we consulted our Gynaec, she said it could be the fibroids acting up. She gave tablets to calm the uterus and protect the foetus - Duphastone (More progesterone) and Duvadilan. That made the nausea rebound.

Nithesh was travelling in March for work. UTiZ is expanding and is now operating in fourteen states in India. Despite all the responsibilities, he still tried to work around from home to spend more time with me. I bought myself a "C" shaped pregnancy pillow and I can't explain what a lifesaver it is. It's so comfortable sleeping inside that. We got a local carpenter to build a shoe rack on our front porch. I wanted to furnish our bedroom and hall soon before the baby arrived but Nithesh wanted to be here while we refurbished. Virgo husbands can be extremely caring but unnecessarily interfering and dogmatic too.

As Amma finally settled back into her normal routine, Achan was contagious with Ophthalmic Herpes. He was soon taken to the hospital by Prashob and shifted to another flat in D Homes as our apartment was already rented out. He stayed there for about two weeks then quarantined upstairs for another few days until he fully recovered.

Acha is the most easy-going person in my life. We have had a very healthy relationship from the beginning. I was closer to him in my childhood as Amma often travelled for her shoots. He'd take me to the parks and the beaches; We'd travel in local transport, have ice-creams and dine out. Somehow he respected boundaries and never questioned me about anything. He made me independent right from childhood and I don't remember ever asking him "Can I?". He allowed me the freedom to make my own choices and learn from the consequences. Having grown up without hearing the word "No" makes me trust my gut and heart. Because everything I ever did was my own choice and I was never forced to do anything anyone else wished. But on the rare occasions when things went wrong, no one stood by me like he did. My strongest pillar! They say the father is the backbone of the family for a reason! Even today I'd say he's the purest soul I have ever known. And this is not because he's my dad, he is just that.

Pregnancy and wedding are the times when everything around you goes for a toss. It could be the most challenging time for the family. Maybe it's all about energies. You are welcoming another soul into your life and the universe performs a little adjustment there.

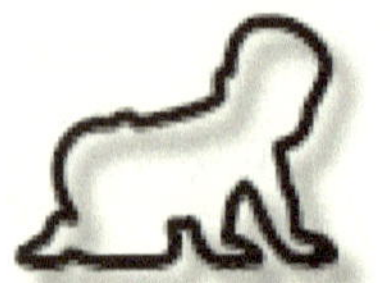

OLD WIVES' TALE - If your nipples appear darker or larger than usual, you are likely to have a boy.

Pregnancy makes your breasts more sensitive than ever. Due to the developments in your milk ducts and changes in hormones to help produce lactation, the shape and size of your breasts could change during this course. This may vary from person to person and has nothing to do with your baby's gender. Your placenta also secretes hormones that increase skin pigmentation. Therefore, your nipples to moles, anything could appear darker due to melanin and it has nothing to do with the gender of the baby.

PREGNANCY MYTHS

CAN I EAT SEAFOOD?

Yes, in fact, the omega-3 fatty acids in fish are highly nutritious for the mother as well as the developing baby. But make sure to avoid fishes that have high mercury content.

DOES EATING SPICY FOOD INDUCE LABOUR?

No, if there was such an easy method, doctors would have had a much easier life.

CAN I WEAR HEELS?

Yes, there is no harm in wearing heels during pregnancy but be careful not to slip or fall as the centre of gravity is now changing and you may lose control of yourself. Avoid wearing heels for a long time as it may increase the chances of back ache.

CAN I DRINK COFFEE?

An occasional sip of coffee or tea or tinned beverages will not affect the foetus but the best move would be to avoid caffeine all nine months. However, if that's difficult, limit your caffeine intake to not more than

200 milligrams per day. This equals to one 8-ounce cup. Research says that caffeine causes the blood vessels to constrict and reduces the blood supply to the foetus. Caffeine acts as a diuretic and can affect the amount of nutrition it gets from the mother. It can also increase heart rate and reduce the absorption of calcium and iron for the mother. Therefore if possible try to avoid caffeinated drinks.

CAN I DRIVE?

Yes, if you are a good driver and are confident about yourself, why not? But make sure that driving does not make you more anxious than you already are. If it is giving you any stress, it may not be advisable.

CAN I FLY?

Yes but in certain cases it may not be advisable so check with your doctor before you make plans. It is safe to fly during the second trimester as there would be fewer complications. One of the concerns of flying is the metal detectors and scanners in the airports which may not be completely safe for the foetus.

SEX IN PREGNANCY?

Yes, it's absolutely safe as the baby is protected in the amniotic sac. As long as you choose comfortable positions and not go too hard on yourself, it is safe.

WEIGHT GAIN IN PREGNANCY

It is ideal to gain 9-15 kgs of weight during pregnancy. However, the number varies depending on several factors.

GAS IN PREGNANCY

This is because everything in the body shifts during this time. The space between the organs changes and the body has a difficult time digesting the food. Pregnancy is a time when you try to eat healthier. So the new addition of gas-forming food items in your diet like lentils, legumes, cauliflowers etc. will make this condition worse.

URINE LEAKAGE IN PREGNANCY

This is because the pelvic floor muscles turn weak due to the hormone changes and because of the uterus putting pressure on the bladder. Urine leakage while sneezing or laughing is a temporary issue.

LEAKY BREASTS

This is normal when the body produces high amounts of prolactin - a hormone responsible for producing breast milk.

VAGINAL DISCHARGE

This is again due to the increase in estrogen levels in the body but if the discharge has a different colour or odour, please report to your doctor.

THE PLACENTA

The placenta is the lifeline between the mother and the baby. It is an organ that develops from the blastocyst inside the uterus after implantation. The placenta provides oxygen and nutrients for the foetus from the mother's blood and carries waste products from the baby's blood to the mother through the umbilical cord. The placenta is also an important endocrine organ that produces hormones which regulate the physiological aspects of the foetus and the mother. The placenta grows throughout pregnancy and separates itself from the uterine wall soon after childbirth. Then the umbilical cord is cut and the placenta too has to be birthed vaginally. In the case of C-sections, it is removed surgically after the baby.

The location of the placenta can influence various aspects of the pregnancy.

There are four types of placenta:

- Posterior placenta: When the placenta grows on the back wall of your uterus, it is known as the posterior placenta. Here, the placenta will be closer to the mother's spine. The foetal activities can be felt during an earlier stage in pregnancy. This location of the placenta also helps to see the ultrasound images more clearly.

- Anterior placenta: When the placenta grows on the front wall of your uterus closest to your abdomen, it is known as the anterior placenta. The foetal movements may not be very clear as the placenta acts as a cushion between the abdominal wall and the baby. In some cases, this placenta makes it quite challenging to see the ultrasound images with clarity.
- Fundal placenta: When the placenta grows at the top of your uterus, it is called the fundal placenta. In most cases, they possess no complications but sometimes by the third trimester, they can lead to a condition called Placenta Previa.
- Lateral placenta: When the placenta grows on the right or left wall of your uterus, it is called lateral placenta. This is a rare location for the placenta and there are a few risks associated with this position. There is an increased risk for Preeclampsia, a breech baby or Placenta Previa.

The placenta can move as the uterus keeps enlarging. So it is possible for them to move upwards and away from the cervix when it is close to 32 weeks and in many cases aid in normal vaginal delivery.

The complications that arise with the placenta are as follows:

- Placenta Previa: This is when the placenta covers all or part of the uterus.
- Placental Abruption: A condition where the placenta separates from the uterine wall during the period of gestation.

- Placenta Accreta: A disorder where the placenta attaches too deeply into the uterus.
- Retained Placenta: This is where a part of the placenta remains in the uterus even after delivery.

Vaginal bleeding, abdominal pain, slow growth of the foetus etc. could be some of the symptoms for a placental disorder. An ultrasound should be able to give the correct picture of the conditions related to the placenta. Your healthcare provider will suggest the best option that is safe for you and your baby.

All placentas serve the same purpose of supporting and nourishing the developing baby. Each pregnancy experience will be unique and the placental location can play a major role in that.

BABYMOON

April flew too soon I guess. Nithesh and I visited Ponneth temple on our wedding anniversary day - April 5th, that's where we tied the knot. We then went to Mararikulam Beach Resort which is a one-hour drive from home. The property was all about breezy coconut grass thatched cottages. It was like living in a reimagined fishing village and we could explore the diverse varieties of flora and fauna. We got a lovely room with a private pool. The private beach was just walking distance from there. We had a heavenly lunch, rested in the room, walked to the beach, played archery, clicked photos, dipped in the pool, had a delectable dinner and slept peacefully till 11 AM to have breakfast.

Reading became my new favourite pass-time and I was addicted to Colleen Hoover's Verity. I know I know! Psycho thrillers aren't the best options to read during pregnancy.

After lunch, we played in the pool again and drove back by evening. I don't remember what went wrong but we got into a detrimental fight while driving back. I was furious. I got out of the car and threw up on the highway and wanted to take a cab back home but he apologised and made me enter the car. We drove back in pin-drop silence till we reached close by. He bought me my favourite Ferrero Roche waffles and took me to our Kadavu to talk about what happened. Kadavu is a riverside near my place. We used to come here during our courtship days in the late evenings. Silent nights under the moonlight. We could only hear the sound of water waves. A serene place where we had never-ending conversations about what kind of future we wanted and a place that gave us multiple opportunities for many sneaky kisses.

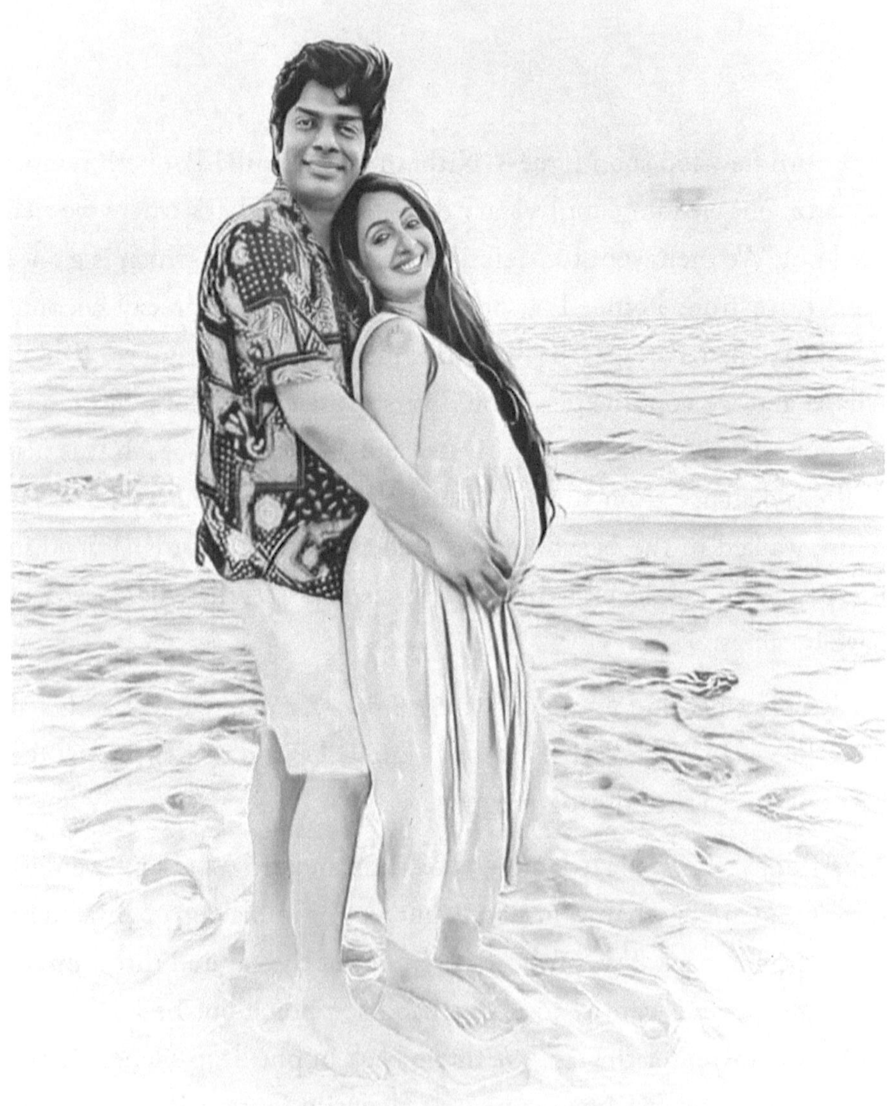

Some fights leave me traumatised even after we solve the issue or even after he apologises a million times. I woke up at 6 AM crying, feeling vulnerable and scared if I'd lose my baby or if shouting could cause hearing problems in the foetus. He hugged me and assured me that we are fine. Even though the fights make me extremely disturbed, I now realise that he's become a part of me and I can't think of a life without him. After all that is marriage, right? Until death do us part... A healthy marriage is about "Us against the world", it's not us against each other. Marriage isn't always a 50-50. Sometimes it's a 20-80 or a 90-10. We need to understand that irrespective of the situation or circumstances, we all have our ups and downs. We all have our good and bad days. We all have our egos and insecurities. Nobody is perfect. When God has blessed us with a little life, it's also our responsibility to stay together in this and to learn to adjust, let go and forgive. Every perfect picture on Instagram has an imperfect story behind it. Perfect couples often fight, cry and argue. The perfection lies in how far one is willing to fight to keep the relationship on, and how far one is ready to compromise to lose the argument just to make the relationship win. It's easy to end things, break the ties and cut off but it's tougher to have difficult conversations, to understand and resolve the disagreements. It's not about how deeply we love but how deeply we hang on to the relationship and how hard we try not to let go.

I do understand that marriages worked in the past even if they were toxic because women adjusted more as they were financially dependent on men. Most of them had no choice other than accepting their husband as their only world. And in today's world, everyone is equally capable despite gender differences. Women are stronger enough to stand up for themselves believing in their rights. But also maybe, just maybe our parents or grandparents had long-lasting marriages because they knew the value of repairing broken things. And we are just so spoilt that we only know to throw things away before it is even broken.

Love doesn't always come easily and knock at your doorstep. It wasn't an easy journey to find him, and it wasn't easy to love him at first sight. We were poles apart different and we still are. Perhaps that's what makes us who we are as a couple. From fiance to enemy to husband to lover and now my best friend, our journey was a rocky road full of surprises. Being married to your best friend is the best thing that can happen in the world but you don't always become best friends with your husband over time. Things worked out better than I ever imagined. Nithesh became everything I ever wished for. And I'm sure he will turn out to be a better father than a better husband.

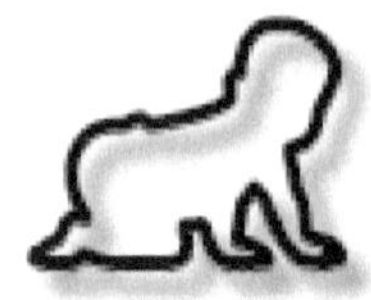

OLD WIVES' TALE - If the length of your linea nigra (the vertical line on your abdomen) starts from below your belly button and extends to your pubic area, it means you're having a girl. If the linea nigra starts all the way from your ribs and extends all the way down, you're likely to have a boy.

This is again related to the hormonal changes in the body and the pigmentation. Many people have a dark linea nigra and for some, it may appear lighter. The length also depends on the extra pigment and has no correlation with your baby's gender. An increase in the production of melanin that causes the facial splotches of melasma also causes the linea nigra. The linea nigra will probably fade back to its pre-pregnancy colour several months after you deliver your baby or may not completely disappear in some cases.

SWOLLEN FEET

Do you suddenly feel like you can't fit into your shoes? Yes, we have all heard about swollen feet during pregnancy but you didn't expect it to be this evident right? Don't worry, it's completely normal.

Due to hormonal changes during pregnancy, the body tends to hold more water than usual. Due to gravity, the extra water tends to gather in the lower parts of the body. The growing uterus puts pressure on the blood vessels, especially the inferior vena cava (IVC) - the large vein on the right side of your body on the back that returns blood from the legs to the heart. So this pressure retains blood and fluids on the legs thus causing swollen feet and ankles. These swollen veins that are travelling from the feet to the heart result in varicose veins. They are usually harmless but can be painful and itchy.

The pressure of the uterus on the aorta and the IVC is the reason why professionals recommend pregnant women to sleep on the side. The left side is recommended due to the position of the organs which are likely to put more pressure on the blood vessels when you sleep on your right.

Swollen feet is a common condition in pregnancy but if you see something unusual, please visit your doctor. Conditions like Preeclampsia, DVT or cardiac diseases also show swollen feet as a symptom.

Limit your sodium intake, reducing caffeine intake, drinking more water and including potassium-rich food in your diet can help with this issue.

A natural home remedy to improve this condition is to soak your feet in warm saline water for a couple of minutes every day and sleep with your feet elevated. Flex your ankles and keep moving your legs every few hours. Do not sit idly in the same position for long and limit your activities that involve too much standing. Getting a foot massage before going to bed also helps.

BACKACHE

Pregnancy can be the most beautiful time of a woman's life but a slight backache can ruin everything. The sudden weight gain and pressure of the uterus can be one of the main reasons. During pregnancy, the body produces a hormone called relaxin that loosens the muscles. This causes instability in the muscles around the spine resulting in pain. Diastasis recti is a condition when the abdominal muscles separate due to being overstretched in pregnancy, making the woman's belly bulge out for years postpartum. This could also lead to lifelong back pains. Sometimes due to the weight of the belly, the spine gets over-arched. This is called lumbar lordosis.

Therefore, a few preventive measures to be kept in mind are as follows. Maintain the correct posture always. Remember to keep your back straight and always use a back support cushion or a maternity belt while working or travelling. Always sit with your spine straight. Get enough rest and don't hesitate to ask for help. Avoid activities that involve a lot of bending or lifting heavy objects.

However, it is not completely under your control. Certain conditions during pregnancy are inevitable.

URINARY TRACT INFECTION

Urinary tract infections are very common in females as compared to males. This is because the tube that drains urine from the bladder - the urethra is shorter in females as compared to males. Also, the distance between the vaginal opening and the urethral opening is very less.

Sexual activities, reduced water intake, high blood sugars, poor hygiene etc. could be the causes of UTI. So drink enough water, maintain your personal hygiene well, be extra cautious while using public toilets and always wash from the urethra to the vagina and not in the opposite direction as it makes bacteria travel into the tract.

Do not treat UTI yourself, always get advice from a medical professional. UTI can be treated easily but if you don't take enough care, it can lead to serious problems.

CAN BABIES HEAR IN THE WOMB?

In the great epic Mahābhāratha, we have heard of Abhimanyu learning his lessons while he was in his mother's womb. There was a time when people ridiculed this concept of a child learning from the womb of a mother. But further scientific developments have made things very clear and modern science says that it is very much possible.

When Abhimanyu's mother Subhadra was pregnant, Arjun told her the secret of entering the Chakravyūh - the military formation. When he was explaining the exit procedure, Subhadra fell asleep, so Arjun stopped there. Hence Abhimanyu in Subhadra's womb learned only the entrance procedure and he never had the chance to learn the exit strategy. This was the reason for his demise at a young age during the Kurukṣetra war. According to Dr. Makoto Sichida, Japanese research says that the right brain is active during gestation. The right brain is the centre for extra sensory perception (ESP). Studies prove that the foetal right brain hemisphere is active and the left brain hemisphere is dormant.

A baby's eyes and ears start forming by the 8th or 9th week of pregnancy. Small bud-like indentations start to form from the baby's head and extend to the neck. These are the ears. They continue to develop rapidly on the inside as well as outside. By around the 18th week, the baby will be able to hear sounds.

The first sounds that your little one hears are the ones created by your body, inside the womb. Though you may not be aware of these, the baby can hear the sound of the mother's heartbeat, stomach digesting the food, lungs breathing air, the vibrations of your voice and so on.

Around the 24th to 27th week, the baby's inner, middle and outside ear develops and the baby begins to respond to sounds from outside the womb. If you want to sing to your child, this is a good time to start doing that.

You must take into consideration that a baby is in the womb under layers of skin and fat and is suspended in amniotic fluid. The outside sounds would be muffled. To understand this, try listening to sounds when underwater in a swimming pool. The world around you will sound muffled. Avoid placing the speakers close to the tummy as these vibrations could disturb the foetus.

It is important to keep the noise level between 50-60 decibels, that is the sound of a normal conversation. It is better to avoid noisy environments during your pregnancy. The noise through speakers in theatres and concert halls could be disturbing for the baby. However, occasional exposure to loud noise will not damage the baby's hearing ability.

It may not be possible to stay away from stress, arguments and fights throughout your pregnancy. Research also says that shouting

and verbal abuse can trigger a neuroendocrine change in the woman, which can decrease blood flow to the uterus. This can be associated with intrauterine growth delays that may well hinder the development of the baby's hearing system. Hence maternal stress due to verbal abuse induced by the partner can cause auditory problems in the baby. So try to avoid negative noise or such situations as much as possible while you are expecting.

MOTHERS IN THE PURĀṆAS

A mother gives birth to a child. But who gives birth to a mother? God? Or does a mother give birth to God?

In a temple, the place where the deity resides is called Garbha Griha. Garbha means womb and Griha means home. Therefore, the temple itself is seen as a female, as a womb - a mother.

According to Sanātana Dharma, Devi is called Kumāri and Māta. Kumāri is not a virgin but a woman who is independent. No man has any right over her. Her hair is untied to symbolise her freedom and hence she is completely liberated. She can be an independent mother and the mother of nature - Prakrti. No one has control over nature.

Characters like Devāhuti, Sīta and Śakunthala are examples of women who have been single mothers - women who raised their children without the help of their husbands.

At the same time, we also come across men who have replaced mothers. Śakunthala was raised by a single father, Kaṇva Riṣi after the Apsara abandoned her. Similarly, when Sīta disappears into the earth, Rām raises the children Luv and Kuśa single-handedly. So the Purāṇas also talk about fathers who played the role of mothers.

We have not only come across positive mothers. Rivalry between greedy and ambitious mothers have been subtly depicted in the Rāmāyana and Mahābhārata. From Satyavati to Gāndhāri, Kunti and Mādri, everyone wanted the best for their children. This was the beginning for many issues. Through Rāmāyaṇa, Kaikeyi's and Kauśalya's story is also well known to prove that mothers can be determined and demanding when it comes to securing the future of their children. But in either case, no one is to be blamed because right or wrong lies in the eyes of the beholder.

Kṛṣṇa was born from Devaki's womb but raised by Yaśoda. So he has two mothers. This story suggests that relationships are not built by blood alone.

Therefore, there are many pregnancy anecdotes and different types of mothers depicted in earlier literary mythological texts.

SĪMANTAM

We performed the traditional rituals of baby shower at home on the 21st and 22nd of April. Dr. Sri Parameswaran Namboothiripadu and his disciples came from Ottapālam. Bhagavati Seva was performed in the evening with a beautiful Kalam. Vāram irikkal was another act that was performed. Mantras from Ṛg Veda were recited for the unborn baby to hear. Sāraswatha homam and japam were part of the ceremony. A ghee with Saraswati mantra chanting is given to the mom-to-be. All parents pray to have a child who's wise and intelligent. These rituals are performed to get the blessings of Saraswati, the Goddess of knowledge.

It was a blessed evening. We wore pink attires and Rakesh clicked our pictures. Friends and family joined us for the function.

The next day we wore green attires in the traditional Thampurāṭṭi style. Gaṇapati homam started early morning. Pumsavanam was an act performed to have a baby boy. As per the old tradition, having a boy was considered more of a blessing than having a girl since boys could become kings and rule the land. Nowadays it is still performed as an act but just to receive a healthy, happy baby. Here the husband asks "Kim Pibathi?" And the wife replies "Pumsavanam" and drinks the holy sweet - Pāyasam. This is repeated thrice.

Sīma is the hairline from the forehead to the end of the scalp. Antham means ending. Fontanelle is known as the Mokṣa Sthāna. One who is a celibate (saint) attires Mokṣa in his life. As per our tradition, married women should not think of attaining Mokṣa. They have responsibilities towards their husband, children and generations to come. It is their Karma. That is why the wedding ceremony commences with the groom applying sindhūr on the bride's forehead. Sīma-antham means putting an end to celibacy.

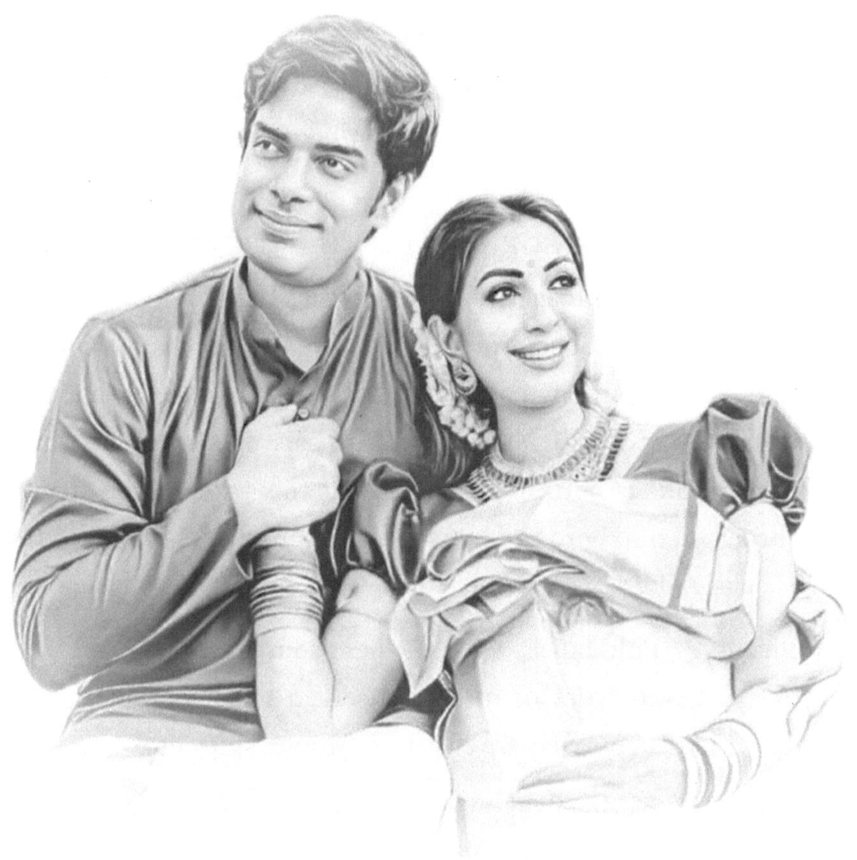

That is why Indian women have a tradition of applying sindhūr on the forehead so that they have a long-lasting married life with a good sex life. "Dhīrgha Sumañgali Bhavaha" they say!

One of the main rituals performed during Sīmantham is where the husband uses the quills of the porcupine to draw a line on the Sīma of the wife. This is said to produce more blood flow in the carrying woman, thus making her happy and healthy and resulting in a better baby.

The ceremonies got over with me singing a Thiruppugazh in Shanmugapriya rāgam in praise of Muruga. I learned the song during my 4th month while I attended music classes with Ananthasree. Music classes during pregnancy kept me engaged a few days a week.

I then wore a black settu-mundu and we had the Valaikkāppu ceremony where aunts of Neptune and a few of my friends joined to give me blessings.

The jingling sound of Kuppivala (glass bangles) is supposed to bring happiness and prosperity to the foetus. That's why the mother is made to wear glass bangles during the seventh month by women in the family. This ceremony is called Valaikāppu. It is an ancient ritual that originated in Tamil Nadu. The Mughals believed that women should wear anklets with jingling bells for the same reason that the sound brings harmony to the foetus. These sounds produce the effect of music naturally.

Puliyūnu or Pulikudi is a ritual where sour water is given to the mom-to-be. Seven types of meals are served to all the guests. This could be various items that are sweet, salty, sour, spicy etc.

Sīmantham or Valaikāppu are ceremonies performed by the pregnant woman's family members at her residence. The husband and his family may or may not take part in the rituals. As per our tradition, the wife then remains at her place until birth and recovery to feel more comfortable and receive more helping hands. However nowadays it all depends on one's comfort and personal choice.

A couple of days later, we had a Śrī Kṛṣṇa Pūja at home performed by Dr. Kiran, the youngest and former priest of Guruvāyūr temple.

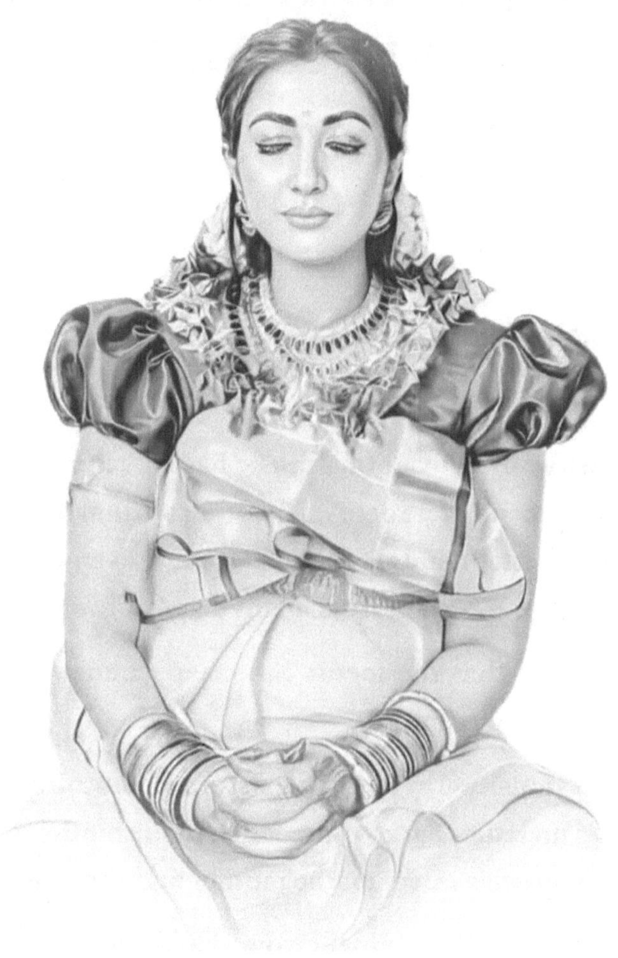

MUSIC, READING AND BRAIN DEVELOPMENT

"Rhythm and harmony find their way into the inward places of the soul"

- Plato, Ancient Greek Philosopher

It is scientifically proven that music has an exceptional effect on the development of a foetus. Music also calms the mother and keeps her in a better mental space. Music is proven to be the easiest therapy anyone can benefit from at any stage of life.

It is believed that the foetus can clearly understand tune and rhythm in the third trimester.

Classical music, rhythmic beats, and soothing music like lullabies and melodies are recommended to the mother which is said to result in a positive effect on the mother and the unborn child.

Exposure to music while in the womb has a cognizant, behavioural and psychological development in unborn babies in comparison to those who did not listen to music while in the womb.

While some instruments bring harmony, certain instruments like Chenda do not produce a soothing effect. Though Chenda is capable of producing complex rhythmic beats, it is called an

Asura Vādya. At the same time instruments like Vīna which is the iconography of Goddess Saraswati, belong to the positive category of Deva Vādya. Listening to a live Veena concert during pregnancy can be refreshing. Similarly, wind instruments like the flute - the instrument of Kṛṣṇa, depict celestial music and are believed to bring divinity through Indian, Chinese and European music.

Indian classical music can have a great impact on the development of the foetus. Research in 2017 proves that women who listened to Kalyāni rāga on a daily basis in the second trimester had a much healthier pregnancy and their babies were born with ideal weight. Kalyāni is the 65th Melakartha Rāga in Carnatic music. The word Kalyāni means "she who causes auspicious things." It is called Yaman in Hindustāni Music and its western equivalent is Lydian Mode.

Similarly, rāga Hindolam of Carnatic music is said to create a soothing and intoxicating effect. The Hindustani equivalent to this raga is Malkaush. It is believed that this raga was created by Pārvati to calm down lord Śiva.

Bhāgeshri rāga found in Carnatic as well as Hindustāni music is said to have a deep effect on the mother and child. It is considered as a midnight rāga that implies situations of yearning by the nāyika for love. This rāga is derived from the Melakartha Kharaharapriya.

Bhairav in Hindustāni is a morning rāga that is said to create a solemn and devotional mood for pregnant women.

Many rāgas create uplifting moods and many create sorrow. Some can make you feel pain and some can make you fear. Indian classical music is deep like an ocean. To understand rāga and tāla, one needs to delve in deeply and do years of Thapasya to attain the knowledge.

Not just Indian music, but music across the world can have positive effects on the mental state of people.

Music is not only therapeutic for babies in the womb. They help them even as they enter the real world. Soft, soothing and relaxing music creates a calm atmosphere for babies and helps them nurture their sleeping patterns. A familiar euphonic tune often works like music therapy. This slow repetitive music will actually slow down the baby's heartbeat and improve deeper and calmer breathing in them.

The English word lullaby is said to have originated from Lala or Lulu sounds made by mothers or nurses to pacify the baby to sleep. Bye is another term which equals to "good night" or putting an end to something. Lullabies are found in every culture in every native language around the world.

Music helps children memorise words, express themselves and understand emotions. Music makes an impact on our ability to connect with one another and makes us involved in empathy, trust and cooperation.

Therefore, music scholars believe that music should be a part of a person's journey at every stage of life.

Similarly, science has proven that reading to the baby in the womb can promote brain activity, early literacy skills and language development. Babies in the womb are learning and understanding the world around them. This continues even after they are born. Babies who are read to often speak more words at two years old as compared to those who aren't read to. While the world is advancing digitally with e-books, it is recommended to engage children with print books. The touch and feel of a print book make children feel more connected to the idea of reading. It is also recommended to avoid screen time completely until two or three years of age.

BRAIN DEVELOPMENT IN THE DIGITAL WORLD

With the rapid advancements in technology, there is so much content out there providing learning opportunities to children. But too much of anything can be harmful.

Some of us as working women or women who need to cook, clean, take care of the elder child etc. may depend on baby cartoons or baby shows available on our phones and tabs to keep our baby or toddler engaged for a while. This at a later stage becomes a daily routine.

More sedentary screen time can lead to less enthusiasm for physical activities which may even lead to poor quality sleep. WHO research suggests that not meeting the physical activity goals in children can lead to several developmental issues and health problems in adolescents and adults.

Studies show that too much screen time during infancy may lead to changes in brain activity as well as problems with executive functioning - the ability to stay focused and control impulses, behaviours and emotions. Longer screen time at one year of age can be significantly linked with autism at three years of age. Back in 1975 when Televisions started becoming popular in India, one in every 5000 children were diagnosed with autism. Now in 2020, with mobiles, tablets, laptops and TVs at our fingertips and Alexa-run homes, one in every 80 children is diagnosed autistic.

The main developmental activities take place in the womb at night when the mother is asleep. So avoid screen time a few hours before bed and a few hours after waking up. Keep your mind relaxed and refreshed with positive vibes, peaceful TV shows, good music etc. Kindly refrain from horror movies, disturbing shows, traumatic scenes and all kinds of negativity for the betterment of the foetus.

ANTENATAL YOGA

"Yoga is the journey of the self, through the self, to the self"

– The Bhagavad Gita

Pregnancy is a time when a woman goes through various physiological and psychological changes and yoga is considered an ancient mind-body practice to maintain mental and physical well-being.

Yoga can be divided into four streams of practice:

- Śakti krama for the youth, children and teenagers - It helps to build strength and flexibility.
- Rakṣaṇa krama for adults - It aids in retaining the abilities of the body and prevents deterioration.
- Ādhyātmika krama for elders. - This method is used for more spiritual practice.
- Chikitsa krama - This can be used by anyone for specific therapeutic conditions.

Yoga for pregnancy belongs to the fourth category where a lot of customisation and modification is made based on each individual's condition and stage of pregnancy. A person's yoga practice changes before conception itself to help prepare for conception. Yogāsana practice should be handled by experienced teachers, especially those experienced in teaching pregnant women.

The purpose of yoga during pregnancy should be to detoxify the mind through prāṇāyāma practices and practice āsanas focused on building flexibility and strength for the pelvis, lower back, hips and legs. The teacher may also choose postures which can help build confidence and mental anchorage for the student to face the changes in the coming months. The very definition of āsana is a posture in which one is stable (sthira) and comfortable (sukha).

The most stable and comfortable āsanas during pregnancy are those practised in seated positions without any strain or pressure on the abdomen. Not all prāṇāyāma practices are suitable during pregnancy. Āsana and prāṇāyāma practices after delivery should also be guided well.

Here are some common āsanas which can be included during your antenatal period:

- Vīrabhadrāsana (Warrior pose)

  It increases the energy levels within the body, gives better balance and builds up the arms, legs and lower back.

- Trikoṇāsana (Triangle pose)

  It helps maintain a balance between physical and mental health, extends and widens the hips, and minimises back pain and maternal stress.

- Baddhakoṇāsana (Butterfly pose)

  It promotes flexibility in the hip and groin area, extends the thighs and knees, reduces fatigue and aids in facilitating smooth vaginal delivery.

- Mārjāriāsana (Cat stretch)

  It helps to ease the stiffness in the neck and shoulders and prepares the spine to bear more weight as the pregnancy advances providing more elasticity to the back.

- Viparīta Karani (Legs up the wall pose)

  It serves to alleviate back pain, advances the blood circulation to the pelvic region and minimises edematous ankles and varicose veins.

- Vajrāsana (Diamond pose)

  This pose assists in increasing the flexibility of thigh, hip and foot muscles and relieves rheumatic pain and heel pain which commonly occurs during pregnancy due to the sudden weight gain.

- Uttānāsana (Forward bends)

  It reduces digestive ailments such as constipation and enhances the digestive process.

- Śavāsana and Yoga Nidra

  They encourage in regulating blood pressure and minimising stress giving more tranquility to the mind and body.

With changes in the body, practice ought to change to accommodate the limitations and focus more on the mind and breath.

The yoga practice should also invigorate the practitioner to find anchorage in an Ishta devata or an entity that one draws strength from and places faith in. For those who connect to sound, Manthrapuṣpam is a powerful Vedic chant from Taittirīya Āraṇyaka (1.22) which celebrates the element "Water" as a powerful primordial force. Traditionally this chant was chanted to pregnant women.

"Personally I have seen this chant work wonders when there are complications in a pregnancy. I have worked with a few students to whom I give only a prāṇāyāma practice along with this mantra with a visualisation and they made rapid improvement in their health." Says Hariprasad Varma, a certified yoga therapist.

Many women who are not used to self-care also take up yoga during their prenatal period to understand their minds and bodies better. Prāṇāyāma practices like Brahmari, Śītali etc. can help silence the mind and nāḍīśodhana can help cleanse the nāḍīs and detox the system.

More than learning about what poses are safe, a pregnant woman should be cautious enough to know what poses need to be avoided.

Yoga postures to be excluded during pregnancy are:

- Naukāsana (Boat pose)
- Chakrāsana (Wheel pose)
- Ardha Matsyendrāsana (Sitting half spinal twist)
- Bhujañgāsana (Cobra pose)
- Viparīta Śalabhāsana (Superman pose)
- Halāsana (Plow pose)

Yogic practice improves and strengthens the immune system, the process of labor and speeds up recovery. But if you have no prior experience with yoga, do not attempt any āsana without the guidance of a teacher.

WEEKLY DEVELOPMENTS IN THE SECOND TRIMESTER

WEEK 14

The baby's arms and legs are growing longer, the liver is producing bile and the spleen is producing red blood cells. For boys, the prostate is developing. Ligament pain may occur at this phase for the mother. A test called Amniocentesis (a sample of the amniotic fluid is taken surgically) is performed to diagnose foetal abnormalities in certain cases.

WEEK 15

The baby's arms and legs are growing longer and the bones are hardening. The eyes and ears are getting close to the final position.

WEEK 16

The baby and the placenta are roughly the same size and fat deposits are building under the skin making the baby more like an adorable newborn. The 50% increase in blood circulation is said to give the mother the "pregnancy glow".

WEEK 17

Baby's auditory developments are starting to take place and cartilage continues to harden. Some may notice an increase in appetite from this week. For some women vaginal secretions may increase. This is called Leukorrhea. Sciatica is a condition where pain travels along the path of the sciatic nerve. Some may also experience needle sensations associated with a leg falling asleep. Applying heat or doing mild exercises may help.

WEEK 18

The baby's nervous system continues to become more refined. Myelin is a protective covering over the nerves. It continues to grow until the baby is one year old. The baby's skin is covered by a greasy substance called vernix to protect it from the amniotic fluid. Backaches and low blood pressure could be a concern at this time.

WEEK 19

In baby girls, the vagina, uterus, and fallopian tubes have settled in the proper place and have several eggs in their ovaries. In baby boys, the genitals are completely formed now. Permanent teeth are forming behind the milk teeth buds.

WEEK 20

The baby is now producing meconium - the first stool. It is stored in the baby's intestines until delivery. In some cases, the baby passes meconium which mixes in amniotic fluid, blocks the airway and injures the lung tissue at the time of delivery. This is referred to as Meconium Aspiration Syndrome. In such cases also the mother may go into an emergency C-section. During this week, skin changes may occur and you may notice changes in eyesight.

WEEK 21

The tongue of the baby is developed and swallowing has increased. White blood cells are being produced and will help fight off infections. Varicose veins, gestational diabetes etc. can be problematic now for the mother.

WEEK 22

Baby's fingernails have grown and the facial features are becoming more defined. The liver is beginning to break down bilirubin and the pancreas is maturing. The baby would be the size of a papaya weighing 400 grams approximately. Swelling may increase for the mother, especially in the legs and there are more chances for UTI now.

WEEK 23

Lanugo, the fine body hair on the baby has darkened and the organs are visible through the skin. Skin issues for the mother may become more prominent now like the linea nigra, stretch marks, melasma etc.

WEEK 24

The baby is probably 12 inches long now. The spine is getting developed and the nerves around the mouth have more sensitivity which aids in the rooting reflex necessary for eating. Back and leg cramps may start becoming more severe for the mother so maintain the correct posture throughout.

WEEK 25

Baby can grasp things with her palm and the hair colour could be more apparent now. The baby would weigh approximately 750

grams. In some cases, the hair may still be white due to no pigment yet. The heart rate may be between 145-170 bpm. By the end of the second trimester, the baby would be as big as a zucchini. Dental problems may start to occur now for the mother. This may be due to the hormone changes that loosen the gums or due to calcium deficiency in the mother.

PREGNANCY GINGIVITIS

Gingivitis is a condition that occurs at the early stage of periodontal disease. Gingivitis is when the gums become red and swollen from inflammation and that may be aggravated by changing hormones during pregnancy. Women are prone to gum diseases and cavities during pregnancy and they can be easily treated. The early symptom could be bad breath. Some may notice bleeding or pain in their gums. Gingivitis is common during pregnancy as the body reduces its ability to respond to plaque bacteria.

It is very important to maintain good oral hygiene while you are pregnant. While visiting the dentist often during this period might be a bit challenging, try to follow home remedies to keep your teeth and gums clean. Brush your teeth twice daily, floss once a day to prevent plaque, gargle with warm saline water, avoid sugary drinks or food and avoid mouthwashes that contain alcohol. Most of the time what happens is that women with nausea tend to avoid the smell and taste of toothpastes which makes the dental conditions worse without proper care.

The foetus takes all its nutrients including calcium from the mother's blood. So if the calcium level in the mother's blood is low, due to reduced absorption from the intestine, calcium is drawn into blood from bone, teeth etc. to maintain the balance.

Gingivitis in worst cases can lead to preterm delivery and if left untreated can lead to tooth loss. This depends on the severity of the condition. Always make sure to check with your doctor before the problem gets worse. In most cases, dental inflammations may go away on their own with self-care and good oral hygiene.

NUTRITION DURING THE SECOND TRIMESTER

The second trimester is when you can relax and relish anything you crave for. There will be comparatively less nausea and less bloating. But have a balanced diet that includes a variety of these groups of foods - vegetables, fruits, dairy, grains and proteins. From the fourth to the seventh month, there will be maximum growth and development in the foetus. The diet during this period should be designed to promote the same.

There's always confusion about whether you should stay vegetarian or non-vegetarian. It totally depends on your beliefs. If you don't eat chicken, fish or eggs, compensate the protein intake with enough lentils, legumes, green peas, hemp seeds, quinoa, peanuts, yoghurt, cheese etc. There are numerous veg protein alternatives.

Calcium intake has to be increased in the second trimester as the growing foetus needs enough calcium for bone development. If you're a fan of paneer or cheese, this is the time to have them voraciously. Dairy products are rich sources of calcium. Leafy greens, badam, dal, channa etc. are also good sources of calcium.

Increasing fat in your diet improves insulin sensitivity and supports the thyroid. Ghee is considered the most divine fat on earth. The addition of ghee to food slows down the rate at which blood sugars climb up. Having good fat helps in burning fat better. Add a teaspoon of ghee to your chapati, dosa, or rice or use it in curries or biriyani. Our ancestors say that rubbing the soles of your feet with ghee before bed prevents constipation and induces better sleep.

Taking a glass of warm water before every meal helps with constipation. Also having the small bananas (Njālipūvan) - a specialty of Kochi, helps in regulating the bowels.

Nutmeg (Jāthikka), rich in antioxidants and minerals helps in improving digestion, better hair and skin, and to reduce blood pressure. Add a pinch of it in milk and drink before bed to induce better sleep.

Add more eggs to your diet as it contains choline which is good for the baby's brain development.

Low mercury fishes are good sources of protein and a dozen vitamins and minerals.

Sweet potatoes are rich in beta-carotene. This naturally converts into vitamin A.

Berries are good sources of vitamin C, potassium, folate and fibre.

Having said that this trimester is the time to enjoy food without much difficulty and restrictions, it's better to watch your sugar intake. This could also be a time that invites gestational diabetes even if you have no such history. So take a pause on that 2 AM ice cream or irresistible urge towards cupcakes and chocolates.

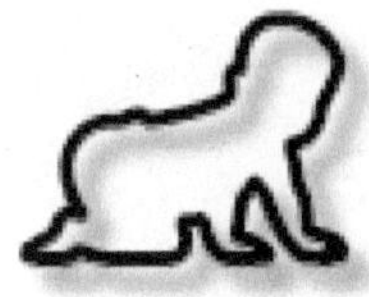

OLD WIVES' TALE – If most of the extra pounds appear throughout your body, especially in your bottom and thighs, it's going to be a girl and if your body doesn't gain any weight but it's just your belly that's growing, it is going to be a boy.

Similarly, if your partner gains weight while you're pregnant, you may be having a girl and if your partner's weight stays the same, you could be having a boy.

Pregnancy weight gain is normal and a must when growing a healthy baby and it completely depends on each individual's body type, pre-pregnancy weight and history of weight gain including conditions like family history of diabetes and many other factors. If your partner and you are linked through mind, body, heart and soul, your partner might be experiencing couvade syndrome. That's when a pregnant person's partner feels the symptoms of pregnancy.

Therefore your or your partner's weight has nothing to do with the gender of your baby.

THE THIRD TRIMESTER

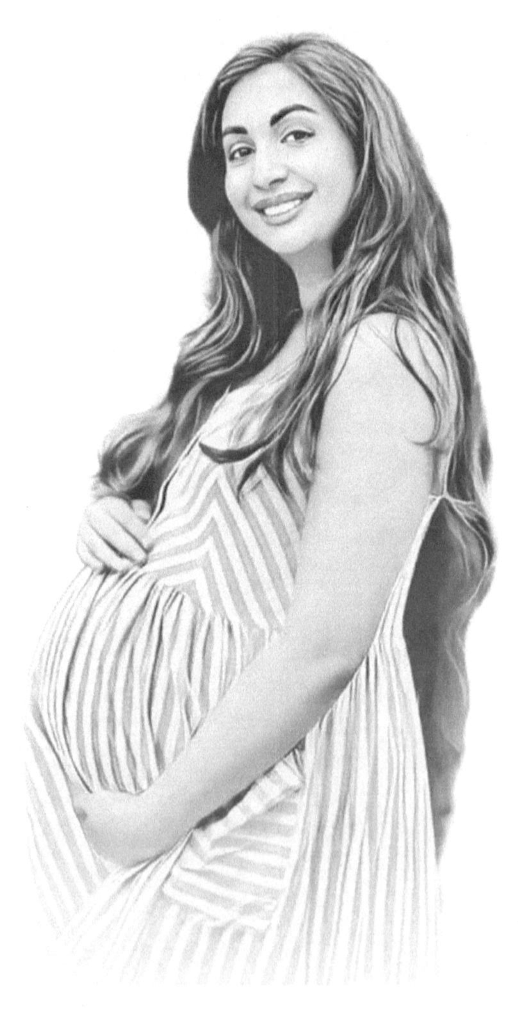

Everything happened too soon. I suddenly lost count of which month we were in and realised that we were always counting behind. I thought I was in the 6th month but I was already 6 months and so many days which means it was almost 7 months. Do you get confused like that? We had to complete the temple visits before completing 7 months. So that was the next thing to be done. Nithesh and I had visited Guruvāyūr in my fourth month before Amma's surgery. We paid visits to Ernakulam Śiva temple and Ravipuram Kṛṣṇa temple during Viṣu. Amma and I visited Pāvakulam, Narasimhamūrthy temple, Pūrṇatrayīśa and Chottānikkara. It felt tiring to hop on and off onto the car now, I have begun to feel very heavy and fatigued. Constant peeing is now a new thing to worry about. Waking up in the middle of the night to run to the toilet isn't all that fun!

The thing that isn't talked about much is the heat during pregnancy. Or is global warming making summers beyond endurance? I rush to the bathroom to take cold showers at least three times a day. The hot flush not only made me sweat, but it made me dizzy throughout the day and night despite the air-conditioning.

If there was one thing I felt throughout my pregnancy, it was my active sex drive. Everything made me feel sensual. And towards the end, it became embarrassing to even talk about it to my husband because anything and everything made me feel salacious.

I felt like I was already due and not prepared with anything. I started panicking. Amma and I started shopping for essentials for the baby. I ordered newborn clothes from H&M on a Wednesday as I wanted to begin the baby shopping on a good day. We got some stuff from First Step and First Cry. Acha also accompanied us once. I bought a lot of maternity pads, creams, baby essentials etc. from Amazon and some maternity wear from Ziva. Nithesh also got some baby essentials from Dubai and the US.

I had the privilege of taking a maternity break and still keep my classes running with the help of three faculties - Nakshatra, Amrita and Krishna. Temple Steps is indebted to their contribution to maintaining the quality of classes even in my absence. It was a blessing to have a job without the hassle of commuting for work, being controlled by a tyrannical boss or anything that was physically or mentally exhausting. I truly enjoyed teaching. Of course, being a performer is physically draining but at this point, everything seems to be working fine.

One day, one of my friends asked me whether I enjoyed teaching or performing more. I honestly did not know. There is a special high while being on stage. As an artist, you get into a trance, where you immerse yourself completely into the music, the rhythm and the character. I once heard a great dance scholar say that when you portray a character, you are touching your inner self that connects with that character out of your perspective. For eg. when you show Radha, you're not becoming Radha, but you are touching the Radha hidden within you. That's how deeply one travels as a performing artist. I don't think anything can replace that joy. But when it comes to teaching, of course, there are days when it feels monotonous with the same Adavus and the same items, yet as a teacher, I feel and experience growth every single day. To see someone start their baby steps to see them become a complete artist who can hold an audience together for a complete recital. The journey is so beautiful. And I think that is tremendously rewarding.

As recommended by Dr. Krishnadas, I started taking baths with Dhānvantharam Kuzhambu more frequently now that we are in the

8th month. Yamini chechi would help me with massaging my back, hands and legs. I would sit for 20 minutes, either listening to music or watching an episode on Netflix and then wash off with Kadalamāvu. These Āyurvedic rituals always made me feel so good and rejuvenated. The muscle cramps at night and the swelling on my feet suddenly vanished.

AMMA OR ACHA FIRST?

When babies start to coo or gurgle, the parents also start eagerly waiting to hear the first magical words - their names. But who comes first? Amma or Acha?

Linguistic experts debate that D's are more difficult to pronounce than M's due to the specific tongue gesture required. So Mamma is often easier than Dadda.

But difficult or not, the first person a child identifies is usually not who we think it would be.

Cross-cultural research shows that the clear winner is the father. American, Asian, European and Indian babies have uttered their fathers' names in their native languages as their first-person words and not their mothers'.

Since mothers are the primary attachment, babies are quite fused to them well into their first year of life. The first separation they see from themselves is from their father. It takes them a couple of months to identify their mother as a different person. For 6-7 months, babies think the mother is a part of themselves and the father is the first person they recognise as someone other than themselves.

ĀYURVEDA DURING PREGNANCY

The Āyurveda concept defines a body as a combination of Vādam (wind), Pitham (bile) and Kabham (phlegm). Humoral pathology explains that the proportion of these humors is responsible for a person's health. The treatment methods can be divided into Śodhana (purification), Śamana (pacification) or Paricharaṇa (preventive measures).

Āyurvedic experts recommend starting an Āyurvedic journey right from puberty. This type of treatment covers all areas of a woman's health such as amenorrhea, painful periods, PCOS, early menopause etc. This type of treatment comes under the category of Sthrī Roga Chikitsa. Pre-bridal treatments are also done to detox the body and uterus which in turn helps in conceiving easily. Śatāvarī Kizhaṅg is a miraculous herb that cures most uterine problems and that's why it is known as a lady herb.

Prenatal care is the primary health care that a woman gets while pregnant. This is called Garbhini Paricharya. The main aim of Garbini Paricharya is to screen high-risk cases, prevent and treat complications and ensure normal delivery with a healthy baby.

According to Āyurveda, the mother should follow Āhāra(diet), Vihāra (lifestyle) and Vichāra (physiological activity) concerning each month. This Garbhini Paricharya can be studied in three parts:

- Māsanumāsika Pathya (Monthly Dietary Regimen)
- Garbhōpaghātakara bhāvas (Activities and substances which are harmful to the foetus)
- Garbhasthāpaka dravyas (Substances beneficial for the maintenance of pregnancy)

During pregnancy, the foetus gets nutrition from the mother through the placenta. Adequate nutrition is needed for proper growth of the embryo and this varies according to the developmental stage of the foetus in each month.

Garbhini Paricharya includes many treatment procedures done by assessing the mother and foetus thoroughly, which helps to enjoy some relaxing time and relieve any discomfort.

During the time of implantation, the body will be more prone to vādam. So special care to balance vādam and strengthen the mother is necessary. Body massages need to be avoided in the first twenty weeks of pregnancy. Vādam causes the fluid in the body to dry up. The application of oil helps in loosening the bones and massages help in toning the uterine muscles. This helps to prevent uterine prolapse and nerve compression which may lead to issues like varicose veins. In Garbhini Paricharya, only Śamana and Paricharaṇa treatments are done. These therapeutic procedures help to increase blood circulation, relieve tension in muscles and melt away stress. It soothes the aching body and eases the process of recovery. It will also help in better breast milk production.

Pāl kaṣāyam or decoctions prepared with milk is advised for the expecting mother to make the pelvis, waist, sides of the chest and back, healthy & flexible and to help the downward movement of vādam (vātānulōmana) to prepare for normal delivery. The most important herb out of them is Kurunthōṭṭi or Bala (Sida cordifolia) which helps the most in preventing abortions.

KAṢĀYAM FOR EACH MONTH

- 1st month - Sida cordifolia, Sanskrit - Bala, Malayalam - Kurunthōṭṭi
- 2nd month - Ipomoea sepiaria, Malayalam - Thiruthāli
- 3rd month - Solanum melongena va, Malayalam - Cheruvazhuthina
- 4th month - Desmodium gangeticum, Sanskrit - Salparni, Malayalam - Orila
- 5th month - Tinospora cordifolia, Sanskrit – Amṛtu Malayalam - Chittamṛtu
- 6th month - Solanum violaceum, Sanskrit - Bṛhati, Malayalam - Putharichuṇḍa
- 7th month - Yava
- 8th month - Clematis triloba, Sanskrit - Laghuparṇika, Malayalam - Perumkurumba
- 9th month - Asparagus racemosus, Sanskrit - Śatāvari, Malayalam - Śatāvari

The Ācharyas explain about the use of enema in the eighth month to relieve constipation and regulate the function of the myometrium during labour.

In most cases, Dhānwantharam Thailam/Kuzhambu is recommended for the garbhini and sūthika as it helps to strengthen the muscles and relieve pain.

Muriveṇṇa helps in relieving muscle cramps as it can lessen water retention in the body. Massaging your feet before going to bed can relieve the pain and relax you for a good night's sleep.

Sahacharādi oil helps alleviate rheumatic ailments like stiffness and muscle cramps. It is also an effective medicine for varicose veins. It can be applied to the lower limbs to treat these conditions.

Your body is now constantly changing and developing to prepare to feed and nurture the baby. Your milk ducts are growing and stretching to produce milk. This could cause your breasts to swell or be more sensitive. Applying oil will help the production of milk and massaging the nipples regularly will reduce soreness during breastfeeding at a later stage.

Applying oil will help mitigate the appearance of stretch marks on the stomach, hips and breasts when used regularly. Massage the stretching skin so that it gets enough moisture and elasticity.

Kerala is famous for its coconuts and that's why it is known as God's own country. Coconut oil has various benefits during pregnancy. Massaging coconut oil on the head is said to promote blood circulation which in turn calms the mother and helps in balancing her mood swings. This also helps in hair growth and hair strengthening. Āmla, Brahmi, Bringarāj, Hibiscus etc. also help in rebuilding undernourished hair.

A tampon of oil may destroy pathogenic bacteria in the vaginal canal and prevent puerperal sepsis. It may also soften and relax the vaginal passage thus helping in normal labour. This is called Yoni Pichu.

Sukhaprasava Ghṛtham is a herbal ghee given to the pregnant mother to assure easy and smooth vaginal delivery. This is given from the seventh or eighth month to calm vātam and pittam. The ingredients in this are upodika rasa, urvaru phala rasa, clarified butter, milk, bhadrika and yaṣṭi. If you're taking any Āyurvedic medicine along with allopathic medicines, seek the advice of the doctor as they may interact and respond differently in the body. Self-medication of any kind is discouraged and expectant mothers with BP, cholesterol or heart diseases should take precautions.

Herbal bath or Vedhu-kuli is prepared out of the kizhi of leaves which helps to balance vāta doṣa. Many leaves like erik, muriñga, etc. are boiled to make Vedh water. The availability of the leaves depends on the season. Dried herbs such as mañjal, athi, ithi, arayal and therāl are commonly used. This is boiled, allowed to cool and poured like a Kaṣāya Dhāra onto the mother. This is an ancient Āyurveda formula that nourishes the skin and restores the body to its healthiest form. During prenatal care, lukewarm water is used and in postnatal care, hot water can be used for śodhana treatment. However, boiling water should be avoided nowadays as most women end up with episiotomy or cesarean stitches.

After delivery, the woman is known as Sūthika. Post-delivery treatments are referred to as Sūthika Paricharya. Only śamana treatments are done for the first fourteen days after delivery.

Later kizhi treatments are done to make the sūthika sweat. With advanced methods like steam baths Śodhana and recovery are also more effective. Pouring hot water on the sūthika or vedh-kuli is known as Pariṣeka. Udaraveṣṭana is tying a cloth belt around the stomach to tighten the hollow space in the body. This helps in shrinking the uterus back to its original size. It also helps in removing vāta doṣa and supports the posture of the back.

During anti-natal care, Garbhini has been advised to avoid factors which produce psychological or physical strain such as Vyāyāma (Exercise), Maithuna (Sexual Intercourse) and Krodha (Anger). However oral medications like Kaṣāyam, Ariṣṭam, Lehyam, Ghṛtam etc. are advised for each woman depending on their health history and these need to be taken only with the advice of a doctor. Antenatal massages have both physical and mental benefits. It relaxes the body and mind and provides numerous benefits to the mother. However, in most cases, pressure massages are not recommended during pregnancy. Prenatal and postnatal massages need to be done only under the supervision of a professional therapist.

I rushed to finish Ranjini's, Veny's and Athira's Varṇams, review Shalini and Upshzara's items for Katchery, see all students once and finish off my classes. There are four Arañgetrams lined up for the next four months once I'm back from maternity break. Arañgetram is a 90-minute solo debut recital of a classical dancer comprising an entire Mārgam, starting from an invocatory piece to a full Varṇam to a Thillāna. It is a significant day in a dancer's life. Rañga Praveśam is the Sanskrit word for Arañgetram. It was tiring but I am so proud I choreographed two Varṇams from scratch without even getting up from my chair. That felt astounding.

I always wondered how I'd manage my classes during pregnancy and it seems like everything always works out if you're willing to try hard. I believe that marriage, pregnancy, raising a baby etc. shouldn't be things that hinder anyone's ambitions. Of course, we need to compromise on many things as women. Even though we protest for gender equality or preach feminism, your pregnancy and your child is going to be your sole responsibility. You may be blessed to have a helping husband who'd wake up at 3 AM for a diaper change or bottle feed, but that's all he can do. Your hormones, your body, your weight, your stretch marks and your mood swings - it starts there! There are numerous things you need to do for yourself. After all, the foetus is developing inside your womb and it is your body that needs nourishment and care. And when you understand that, you will be mentally preparing yourself for all the responsibilities. Do not ever bring a child into your life to save your marriage. Do not have a child due to societal pressure. Do not have a child because you are getting older. Do it only if you're hundred percent sure you want this and only when you are hundred percent ready. It's not just about managing the pregnancy or postpartum. It is a lifelong commitment for which you may or may not have support. Because you don't know what's going to be in store for you tomorrow. Prepare yourself way ahead and that way you would complain less and have a more positive approach towards this mommy game. Never complain about the things you couldn't do because you had a baby. Never curse the child for the opportunities you lost, for the time you lost. The child did not ask to be born. It was your decision and your choice. Motherhood should be riveting and beautiful and should never feel like a chore.

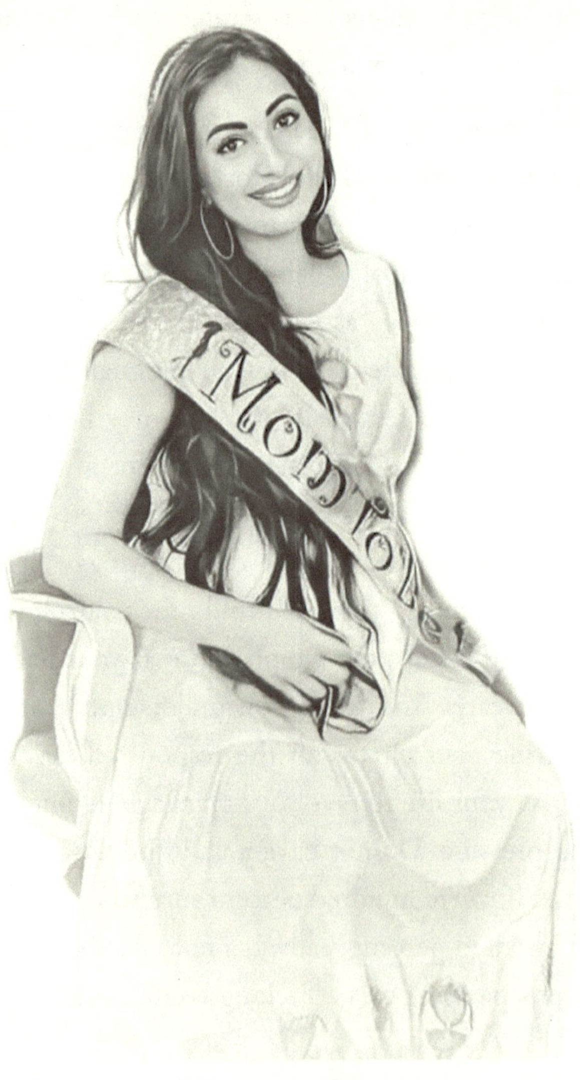

My students gave me a surprise Baby Shower at the end of May. It was really sweet of them. Many online students had sent video wishes too. Having dance students is always like having sisters. From my haldi night to wedding arrangements, lighting diyas on Diwāli or celebrating our birthdays, my dance babies always had my back. Amma always said that dance classes should have a festive vibe and should never have the atmosphere of pale gloomy 10th board classes. The main goal should be to dress up, show up and have lots of fun. Of course, the training is intense, with lots of theory to delve into, complicated talas that drive you mad and never-ending rehearsals before performances. The idea should be to approach art in an artistic way because dance is not a sport, it is a cultural way of living.

Nitya finally came back to me and apologised for her wrongdoings. Like birds, they fly away, but sometimes they come back to their nests.

BHARATANĀTYAM DURING PREGNANCY

"My dance is the truest expression of who I am, because in it, all that is best in me is crystallised.

When I dance, I feel I am at once a poet, a painter and a singer. But ultimately for me, dance is a prayer with my entire being – a transforming experience, a joyous celebration of life."

– Padma Bhūṣaṇ Smt. Alarmel Valli

There is no research that proves or denies that Bharatanāṭyam has benefits on your pregnancy. However, studies show that mild movements of dance can keep the mother and the unborn baby healthy and stress-free. It is hard to stay motivated to be active when gravity changes begin to take effect on your body. There will be less bloating, better energy levels, less constipation and fewer backaches if you try to stay active during pregnancy. Dancing helps you stay well-balanced and coordinated with your body. It releases stress and tension for you and the baby. Dancing is also a great way to bond with your unborn child.

Dancing is indeed an extension of yoga. The mind-body practice is relevant when it comes to dance. The human body goes through many substantial and psychological changes during the prenatal period which are reversible after delivery with proper care. Fatigue and exhaustion are common due to the increase in oxygen consumption during this period. Cardiovascular changes such as an increase in blood pressure, changes in heart rate and pedal edema may happen in the body. Muscular and ligamentous laxity due to hormonal changes and foetal growth takes effect. The centre of gravity changes with the growing belly and hence posture imbalances can occur during this phase. The mother may feel insecure and nervous. Depression and loss of appetite may arise.

Bharatanāṭyam is one of the oldest forms of Indian classical dance. It is a combination of Nṛtta (dance) and Nāṭya (enactment). Most Adavus in Bharatanāṭyam are performed in Araimandi - The half squat position. This not only helps with strengthening the hips and thighs, but it also has major benefits on the health of a woman's uterus. The pelvic floor is much more stronger in a dancer's body compared to a regular body.

All the Adavus in Bharatanatyam are performed by holding the core tight. The right kind of balance is maintained throughout this art form. Adavus like Maṇḍi, Sarikkal etc. which are performed with the full squat jumps also require a lot of core strength. Muzhumaṇḍi (full squat position) is one of the greatest hip flexing activities.

The spine is always straight in Bharatanāṭyam. Even when you perform bends, it is to be kept in mind to hold the spine straight. A slanting line, a perpendicular line, a horizontal line - the line is to be maintained. This is all in terms of Nṛtta. That is just the physical aspect of dance. To be true to your dance, one needs to internalise the art form.

Do not attempt Bharatanāṭyam during pregnancy if you have no prior experience. However, if you are a dancer, check with your doctor before you include dance as part of your pregnancy routine. Avoid Adavus that involve jumps like Uthplavana or those that involve fast spins. Avoid anything that's strenuous and tiresome during pregnancy.

Apart from the physical benefits, dance also keeps a woman mentally in a better place. Listening to Carnatic music will have a soothing effect on the foetus. Especially those with mṛidañgam beats. Different rāgas set different moods for the mother and the baby. Listening to good jathis should also have a positive effect on the foetus. Overall the coordination between the mind and body can work out well when practising Bharatanāṭyam because everything revolves around rhythm.

"Everything in the universe has rhythm,
everything dances"

- Maya Angelou

There are four happy hormones that we commonly come across. Dopamine, Oxytocin, Serotonin and Endorphin. Would it be difficult to believe that all the four are released while performing Bharatanāṭyam? The dance form can have numerous benefits for the mother and the baby.

Dopamine is the rewarding chemical. It is released when you accomplish a task and feel satisfied. It could be little wins that make you happy. Self-care activities, finishing a meal, completing work etc. could feel rewarding. Dancing for ten minutes could also be rewarding. Bharatanāṭyam releases dopamine.

Oxytocin is the love drug. It is released when you hug your loved one, pet your dog or hold a baby in your hands. As humans, we crave for love even if no one openly accepts it. Love in some form is crucial for our survival. Indian classical dance forms aim at communication through the body. The forms like Bharatanāṭyam or Mohiniyāṭṭam that we practice today originated from the text Nāṭyaśāstra. Nāṭya means acting. That is drama. Nāṭyaśāstra is the text on dramaturgy. Bharatanāṭyam is an art form that extensively uses different contexts of love. The Nāyika who's waiting to make love to her husband or the mother who cannot stop cuddling with her child. Performing such an act brings the dancer into a state of trance where she herself feels the love. Because to act is to feel. It is the journey of an artist into her deeper self. Hence oxytocin is released.

Serotonin is the mood stabiliser. Exposure to the sun, meditating and calming the mind, spending time in nature, enjoying a relaxed day at the beach etc. could produce this hormone which makes anyone content. Bharatanāṭyam like yoga is one of the best forms of exercise not only for the body but for keeping the mind focussed too. Bharatanāṭyam is not just Nṛtta (dance), it includes Bhāva (Expression) and Rasa (Aesthetic Experience).

Endorphin is the pain killer. Exercising, laughing, playing games etc. could release endorphins. Bharatanāṭyam being a form of heavy physical activity releases enough endorphins to keep your mind refreshed.

Therefore Bharatanāṭyam is one of the activities that triggers the release of all such happy hormones at once. It is important to stay fit and happy both mentally and physically during pregnancy and pursuing your favourite art will only be helping you and your developing foetus. But if you are a person with no prior experience in dance, this won't be the best time to start. Always consult with your doctor before attempting any new activity. Make sure to avoid challenging movements that add more difficulty to your body.

The goal here is not to get better at dancing, it is about enjoying the movements and being active during gestation. So take it slow and make sure to listen to your body. If you feel dizzy or feel any pain, stop immediately. Refrain from doing anything that makes you feel uncomfortable. Remember to stay hydrated and filled with nutrients during these activities.

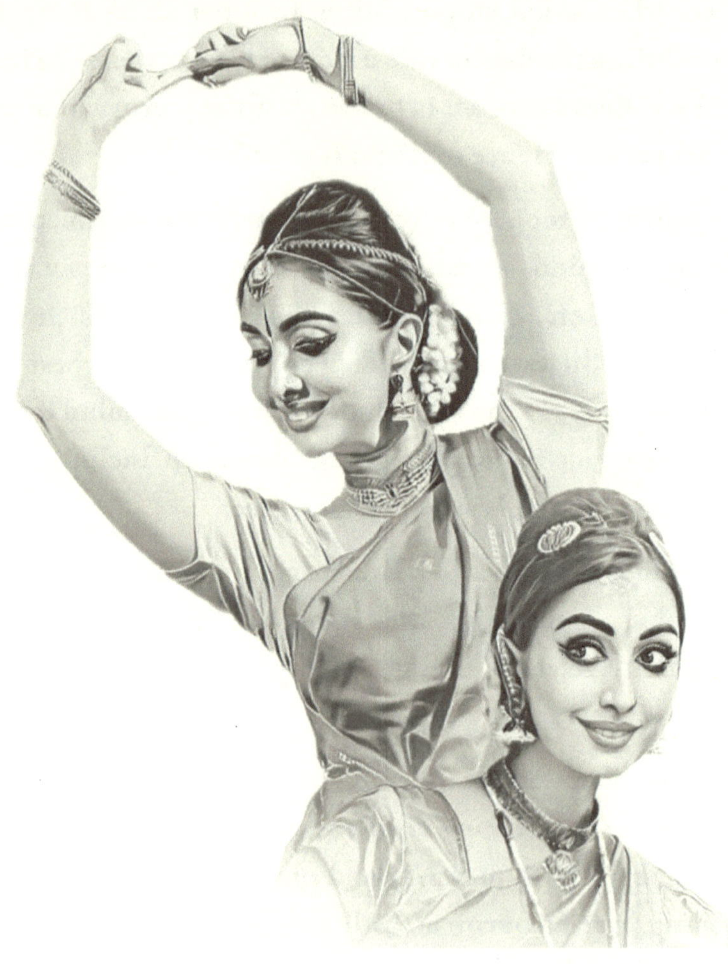

The ancient texts on dance or dramaturgy do not talk about the physical benefits of dance and there is not enough research that scientifically proves how much dance contributes to a woman's health.

But from my personal experience dance does cure a lot of your infertility problems, PCODs, PMS, and many such ailments women are affected with. Most dancers I know have had normal child labour. One classic example is my mother who had a painless normal delivery almost 3 decades back when epidural or such advanced medical care was not yet available in India. She still says she did not experience any pain during her delivery. It's hard for many of us to believe. A lot of my students with irregular periods and PCOS have told me that they now have regular periods after a few months of dancing. Some of them with excruciating periods have also told me that it hurts less now and they have stopped taking medication. A lot of my students have gotten pregnant and stopped dance classes over the past few years. Some friends made fun of me by asking if I was running a fertility clinic or a dance class. But what made me the happiest is that one of my students after trying for eight years - 4 years of treatment after which her doctor said she could not conceive and was asked to try other options, naturally conceived after joining my class online for about a year. It's pure magic!

Bharatanāṭyam helps you with everything you need. I couldn't be happier hearing things like this. It feels like there's a larger meaning to the dance. It is indeed a universal gift.

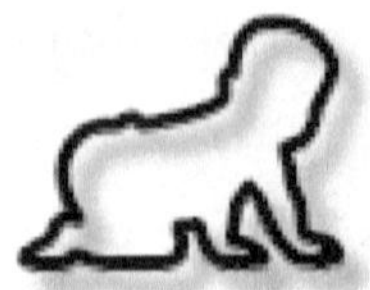

OLD WIVES' TALE - If you consume foods such as eggs, meat, almonds, spinach, salmon, legumes etc. the baby will become intelligent.

Intelligence does not just magically develop from food. Of course, there are nutritious values for these foods and they help in the baby's brain development but intelligence depends on many other factors. So eating right to make the baby smart is simply a myth.

We had a final scan on June 2nd. The doctor said the baby is already 2.5 kgs and I need to control my sugar intake as the baby may grow larger and it would be difficult for a vaginal delivery. The baby is now kicking and moving a lot inside the tummy. This foetus is super-active during the night and sleeps during the day. But I guess all foetuses are like that and that's why they take a while to get adjusted to the real world timings once they come out of the womb.

Crying became a regular thing. And I know it's the mood swings but I'd often cry for the most ludicrous things - like when I'm hungry or if I feel heavy and tired to walk to the bathroom. Everything felt hard, like even bending to pick up things or turning sides while lying down. Are things ever going to get back to normal?

The thing that no one told you about adulting was that everything hurts and this is not just during pregnancy. Never-ending bills, standing up for yourself, being responsible for your loved ones, fighting for your relationships to maintaining your emotional well-being; There is just too much load on us. We were not prepared for this. What did 6-8 hours of school teach us for twelve years? Trigonometry and Algebra that never come of use? Or physics, geography and chemistry? Mental health, sex education, social responsibilities, time management, crisis management etc. were important to have been taught. Perhaps then we wouldn't have been a depressed generation fighting for success. Stop with all the over-positive quotes - She's unstoppable, she's fierce and brave! NO!! She's vulnerable, fragile and broken. She needs help. The global health data exchange confirms that 350 million people are suffering from depression in 2022. There are no super moms, they all go through postpartum blues. There's no perfect daughter, wife or girlfriend. There's nothing shameful about admitting that you need help. Pregnancy mood swings are real, postpartum mood swings are anarchic. Mood swings during your menstrual cycle and menopause are also extremely tough. It's humane! It is normal. You don't have to be ashamed for "crying like a girl". You are a girl and you have all the right to cry. Venting will help and suppression can kill.

I have finally selected 4 boy names and 4 girl names - Now it's Nithesh's turn to select one. We had spoken about this months back. He will only select from the options I gave him but the final selection will be his! The clock is now ticking!

During the time I got pregnant, four of my other students had also conceived. Krishnaja (Dubai) gave birth to a baby girl, Sandra (Trissur) had a baby girl, and Rojna (Calicut) had twin boys. Next is me and then Manasa (US) will be having a boy. I felt like we formed a mini community now. Sometimes we message each other about our cravings, moods, and bodies and sometimes we educate each other with the little information we collected from the internet or elders.

SEX DETERMINATION

Prenatal sex determination is illegal and a punishable offence in India as per the Act passed by the Indian Parliament in 1994. WHO has stated that selecting the sex of the foetus raises serious moral, legal, and social issues. Sex selection or the modification of the natural sex ratio will lead to a gender imbalance in demographics. Some countries/communities, still continue to terminate the female foeticide. Thus revealing the sex of the baby is not legal in many countries as sex stereotypes towards women and devaluing females continue to take place around us.

The WHO defines sex selection as the practice of using medical techniques to choose the sex of the offspring, which encompasses several practices including selecting embryos for transfer and implantation following IVF, that can result in selectively terminating a pregnancy.

The latest high-technology gender selection methods are PGD/PGS (Preimplantation Genetic Testing). But at least six nations have already banned the use of gender selection technologies, and those are Australia, Canada, China, India, and the UK. However, the older methods of gender selection like ultrasound or amniocentesis plus abortion, and infanticide continue to be practised worldwide despite bans.

I had doctor appointments on June 15th, and June 24th and a scan on June 28th. According to the doctor, July 5th is the date for admission if I don't get any pain before.

Amma and Chechi started seeing the Malayalam stars on each date figuring out which could be more beneficial for the child's future. But whatever is said or done, if normal delivery is the option, no one can predict the future of the new avatar.

Packing the hospital bag can be a bit overwhelming. You don't know what to buy and what not. But it isn't all that taxing as you think. Anything and everything you need is available in the stores nearby if you're staying in a city. Most of the time women end up buying a lot of unnecessary items due to the excitement and perplexity.

HOSPITAL BAG CHECKLIST

Packing can be overwhelming so here's a quick checklist in case you're wondering what things need to be carried.

- Administrative items like medical records, insurance papers, ID proofs, cash and credit cards. It is better to decide on your baby's name, exact spelling and all details to be given on the baby's birth certificate. The procedure of registering the birth certificate at the hospital is easier than doing it later. The last thing you would want after delivery is to have confusion on documentation. Discuss this with your partner before and fix it.
- Clothing for the mother - maternity panties, nursing bras, maternity nighties. Front open dresses or zip wear will be very comfortable to help with regular feeds for the baby.
- Toiletries - your usual soap, shampoo, toothpaste etc. and maternity sanitary pads. They are bigger than the usual pads and hold more blood. Breast pads may also be of use. Get a nipple crack cream or simply use coconut oil from day one. You can also try using a nipple shield if it is too painful. Carry your stretch marks cream. Yes, the beauty hacks need

to start off in the hospital itself. Most importantly, the abdominal belt. The sooner and longer you wear it, the faster it helps in shrinking the uterus to its original size. A three-piece postpartum belt or one that covers the whole abdomen will be advisable. Check with your doctor before you wear it because each body is different.

- Keep yourself entertained. Meditate, pray, chant or simply listen to music, watch your favourite shows or engage in a book. Delivery time can make you really anxious so keep yourself engaged.
- Baby clothes, burp cloths, swaddle towels, blankets, diapers, and mittens.
- Your bystander's bag. That could be your mother, husband, friend or sibling. Whoever is taking charge of hospital duties, they better be prepared to deal with difficult nights. Even with nurses nearby, the first night with the baby can be extremely exhausting.

That's about it I guess. The rest of the things you can buy once you're home. By then you will have a clear idea of what exactly you need.

WEEKLY DEVELOPMENTS IN THE THIRD TRIMESTER

WEEK 26

The baby is now about 13 inches long. The eyes have finally opened and retinas are forming. The baby may be moving a lot in the uterus and the mother may enjoy it though some women experience discomfort. Constipation could be an issue during this time.

WEEK 27

The baby is growing bigger and finding it difficult to move around in the uterus. Braxton Hicks contractions may begin for the mother. It may not be painful but it can be jarring.

WEEK 28

Rh factor is a protein found on the surface of red blood cells. The majority of the population are Rh positive but if the mother belongs to the smaller group of Rh negative, she will receive a special Anti D shot during this time. This will be repeated at 34 weeks and during delivery.

WEEK 29

The baby is now around 1 kg weight and the baby's head is now in proportion. The baby would now be the size of a cabbage.

WEEK 30

From now on the baby can turn at any time into the head-down position. The baby's brain is expanding and controlling breathing and maintaining body temperature. The mother may feel more fatigued.

WEEK 31

Some babies may have good hair by now. The eyebrows and eyelashes may also have been formed. The mother may be asked to count the number of kicks she feels to make sure there's good foetal activity in the womb.

WEEK 32

The baby is now about 16 inches long and 1.5 kg. Braxton Hicks contractions may occur more frequently. Researchers also say that at this stage babies can dream in their sleep. Aww!

WEEK 33

The baby's skull and skeleton are complete and the amniotic fluid has topped out its maximum level. The immune system is also developed by the antibodies passed on by the mother. Leukorrhea may be increasing and if it is accompanied by redness, burning, itchiness or anything unusual, consult your doctor. 3D ultrasound can give a clear picture of the foetal position at this point but some hospitals do not recommend this unless there is a complication.

WEEK 34

The baby must be 2 kgs and may be blinking and responding to light. The mother may feel itchiness in the belly which is completely normal. But if there are red patches or if it spreads to other body parts, it could be PUPP (Pruritic Uricarial Papules and Plagues). Another problem is due to the dysfunction of the liver called Cholestasis. Both can be treated with medication.

WEEK 35

The baby's kidneys are fully developed and the liver is fully functioning. Babies born after this week are most likely healthy without any serious complications. The mother may experience lightning or baby-dropping symptoms.

WEEK 36

The baby is growing with an increase of 200 grams every week. The doctor will now start cervix examinations every week to check if the mother is dilating. Some women may notice symptoms, some may feel nothing. So doctor appointments may become more frequent from now on.

WEEK 37

The baby is officially full-term now and is most likely to weigh more than 2.5 kg. Losing the mucus plug can happen anytime now. If you notice bloody discharge, immediately call your doctor.

WEEK 38

The baby's organs are fully developed and functional. The baby's first bowel movement is in the making. If the baby passes meconium,

the mother may run into an emergency. The mother's breasts may leak colostrum sometimes a few days before the baby is born.

WEEK 39

The average baby weighs 3.5 kg and would be 18-20 inches long. Baby nails would be long now. If the water has broken, labour will begin soon. If it doesn't start in 24 hours, the mother may be induced due to the risk of infection. Water breaking can sometimes be a slow leak and in some cases a sudden rupture.

WEEK 40

Pregnancies are not allowed to continue beyond 40-41 weeks as the placenta will not be able to support the baby past this time. Labour is induced through medication in such cases concerning the well-being of the mother and baby. The baby's heart rate remains between 130-170 bpm during the time of delivery.

NUTRITION DURING THE THIRD TRIMESTER

The growing belly makes it difficult to have full meals now. Try to cut down the meals into smaller portions and consume them at regular intervals. Drink enough fluids and keep munching healthy snacks in moderation during this time. The diet in the final stages of pregnancy should be to help the woman withstand the strain of normal vaginal delivery and to improve lactation.

Turmeric is a natural ingredient used for multiple purposes. It's a natural anti-inflammatory medicine and helps with swelling which is a common problem during pregnancy. Studies show that it has many major benefits on the body and brain due to its active compound curcumin. Having a glass of milk with turmeric helps improve your immunity and reduces the chances of allergies due to its antioxidant properties. Include turmeric in your curries as a natural ingredient and avoid using turmeric supplements. Some studies also say that turmeric works as an anti-depressant.

Now is the time to stock up with more protein. The easiest lentil that you can digest is dāl. It is rich in folic acid, vitamin B6, minerals and proteins. Mooṅg dāl is the least gas-forming and reduces the risk of diabetes, high blood pressure and cancer.

Include rice as an important meal in your diet. The resistant starch in rice helps the gut bacteria. Spiritually the grain of rice symbolises health, growth and prosperity according to the Indian tradition. Your local delicacies like kañji, curd rice, rasam rice, dāl chāwal etc. are not only divine and delicious but also super easy to digest.

Keep a control on sweets and other sugary items as it may increase the weight of the foetus in an unhealthy manner and gestational diabetes is still a threat to the mother.

Ammayi's natural home remedies

Boil a glass of water with a pinch of fenugreek seeds (Uluva) and have it on an empty stomach every morning. This not only lowers your sugar levels but also helps in the production of milk after delivery. It can be consumed as kañji when boiled with rice too. Fenugreek helps in weight loss and reduces bloating. However, having large amounts may lead to a drastic drop in sugar levels which may not be advisable.

HEARTBURN

A cup of cold milk will help with heartburn in the middle of the night. In fact, drinking anything cold can help relieve this irritation - juice, iced tea, coconut water, buttermilk, lassi, milkshakes or simply a glass of iced water. Now that the uterus is growing in a size much larger than its usual size, the space for other organs seems to get compressed. The growing uterus tends to press against the stomach and that produces acid refluxes. Spicy food or heavy meals can trigger heartburn. So avoid heavy meals, especially at night and consume food in moderation.

PERINEAL MASSAGE

The area of tissue between the vaginal opening and the anus is the perineum. That is your pelvic floor. It attaches itself to the reproductive organs, bowels and bladder.

Perineal massage is the act of stretching and manipulating the vaginal tissue using a finger or two to stretch and prepare for vaginal delivery. This helps in the smooth movement of the baby's head through the vaginal canal without tearing or pain.

Research says that about one in fifteen women who do regular perineal massage do not require an episiotomy or experience tear that requires stitches. Even if the massage doesn't prevent tearing it reduces the need for stitches by 10 percent. Therefore massaging the perineum reduces the intensity of tearing to a great extent.

Experts suggest that it is good to start a perineal massage somewhere between your 34th and 36th week. You may follow this routine daily or three to four times a week. No matter how often you do it you only need 5 minutes a session to see possible outputs.

You may use a variety of oils like sunflower oil, coconut oil, olive oil or vaginal lubricants to perform the perineal massage. Make sure to wash your hands and cut your nails to keep the vaginal area clean and away from infections.

Please note that this does not guarantee that you'll not tear or wouldn't require procedures like an episiotomy but it can help overall to make the natural birthing a better experience.

End of June, it started raining. Monsoon is just around the corner and I always have mixed emotions during this time. Edavappāthy, that's what it's called in Malayalam - The southwest monsoons! The name of my debut Malayalam film was called Edavappāthy, directed by the late Lenin Rajendran. The movie was so close to my heart. It hits my heart like a cool breeze when I think of the lovely memories and how much I enjoyed working on that film. I played dual roles, one as a modern girl and one as a period character - Vāsavadatta - a fictitious character from Kumaran āsan's poetry Karuna. The renowned actress Manisha Koirala played my mother's role in the film and it was beautifully shot by the ace cinematographers Madhu Ambat and Hari Nair. Edavappāthy also makes my heart heavy like the dark clouds that are about to pour because the commercial outcome of the film did not pay justice to my hard work.

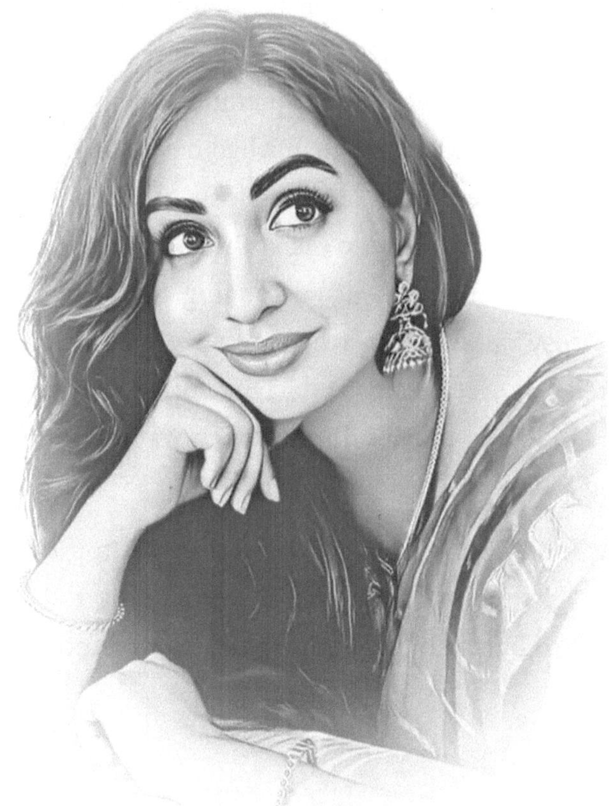

Yes, monsoon has so much to convey like the emotions in my head. The melancholy of vacations getting over. I always hated school - from LKG to 12th standard. Raincoats and umbrellas took up all the space in classrooms. The school bus had a foul smell due to the wet seats and wet socks that some kids wore. There was a June when everything around me looked colourful for the first time when I fell in love. The rain made me sing and dance. Life felt like a movie where there was background music by A R Rahman all the time. I felt like we moved in 55 frames, slow motion. There was a time when I moved to Mumbai - New friends, new home and when adulting felt like a slap on the face. I'd get drenched in the local transport I took to work and I was getting paid in peanuts. Empty purse and rainy nights contemplating whether to order pizza or satisfy myself with leftover bread. A heartbroken June when I looked at the rains and felt like nature was weeping for me. I have been the loneliest, deprived of love. A rainy day in Paris that spoilt my chances of clicking chic holiday pictures. The day I thought that a bad day in Paris was still better than a bad day in any other part of the world. Then there were COVID-19 rains right after my engagement when Nithesh and I couldn't see each other. We were stuck in different cities and the government kept postponing the release of lockdown. And then a cosy rainy season when we were just married. Mummy's home-cooked food, ice creams and Mangalorian delicacies we enjoyed along with music and movies on the couch watching the season pour through our windows.

But this monsoon will be special and it will top the list. It's like waiting for a gift to arrive. And he or she is going to be ours forever. We can't wait to hold our little munchkin in our hands.

OLD WIVES' TALE - Drinking saffron milk every day will help in delivering a fair-skinned baby.

There is nothing anyone can do to change the complexion of the baby. This is genetically decided. Dark-skinned babies have more melanin in their bodies than fair-skinned ones. A baby's eye colour, hair colour, skin colour etc. are decided at the time of conception and no food the mother eats is going to change that.

BREAST-FEEDING

Nobody has to tell you that breastmilk is the best milk. You might have heard that from every corner of the world. But what you're about to discover is that breastfeeding is hard work. You need to keep your body well-nourished to keep your milk supply flowing. Food was your fuel and now your food is the fuel for your baby. There are many easy-to-cook recipes that help you increase your milk supply. It's best to start including these in your diet during the eighth or ninth month of pregnancy and continue them for the next couple of months after delivery. Make sure you don't restrict yourself on your food intake while breastfeeding. You may feel hungrier than ever postpartum while feeding because you lose about 300 calories per day. Make sure to compensate for this by eating healthy. Isn't it the best part that breastfeeding helps you lose weight naturally and much sooner than you expect?

Uluva (fenugreek) water or uluva kañji is a great source to increase your lactation.

When the right amount of minerals is not received from the diet, it is borrowed from your bones. Loss of bone density may lead to a condition called Osteoporosis. Mutton soup made of bone broth is rich in calcium, magnesium and phosphorous. Hence it prevents this condition. It contains glucosamine and chondroitin that helps reduce stiffness and joint pain. The relaxin hormone loosens everything and bone broth post-pregnancy helps in strengthening joints and returning things to normal. Bone broth is rich in gelatin and collagen which is a beauty nutrient that helps in good skin, hair and nails.

Pumpkin spice smoothie - Mixing pumpkin puree, mango, carrot and coconut milk in a blender along with cinnamon and nutmeg powder is a healthy lactation-boosting creamy smoothie.

Oats in all forms help in lactation. Boiling oats with milk and sugar can be a creamy sweet semi-solid drink. Overnight oats soaked in milk or water along with fruits and nuts is a great idea for a quick breakfast. Oats cooked in water with salt and spices like kañji is also a good source for milk production.

Moringa leaves are considered as a natural Indian medicine to treat various diseases. It is an antioxidant which protects the liver and reduces cholesterol. Moringa increases milk production and so expecting mothers are made to have ghee rice with crushed moringa leaves for lunch.

Ghee rice with shallots (Cheriya uḷḷi) is not only a great source of milk, it is one of the tastiest recipes during pregnancy and postpartum. Deep fry shallots in ghee until golden brown, add cooked rice into the pan and mix well. You can add cashews and spices and garnish with coriander leaves to make it more interesting like a mini version of biriyāni.

Milk produces milk. Most of the time women are made to drink milk and have nutritious food during pregnancy. But this isn't followed during postpartum. It is either because many are trying to shed their weight or simply because now all the attention is on the baby. In order to keep your baby healthy with good feed, the mother needs to pay attention to her calcium and protein intake. You need enough calcium to produce milk. So enjoy all the dairy options available around you - yoghurt, cheese, paneer etc.

Salmon is rich in protein, vitamin B12, omega 3 and vitamin D. It is great for breastfeeding mothers as it contains a large amount of DHA, a fat that is important for the development of the baby's nervous system. The best part is that it also tackles postpartum depression. Baked salmon and sardines are good for increasing milk supply.

Eggs are good sources of protein and calcium. Omelettes with healthy fats like avocado, cheddar cheese and some greens would be a great recipe for a nutritional boost.

Chicken soup with some turmeric and fresh veggies is not only yummy but it also gives your body enough energy to breastfeed.

BENEFITS OF BREASTFEEDING

There are numerous benefits of breastfeeding for the mother and the baby. The mother will be transferring antibodies and necessary nutrients to the baby through breast milk thus increasing the immunity of the baby. The first milk which is a watery yellowish discharge - colostrum - is known as gold because it has everything needed for a healthy baby. Breast milk helps fend off colds, flu, and infections and reduces the risk of sudden infant death syndrome (SIDS). Years of research also suggest that breastfed babies are less prone to asthma, digestive issues and obesity. Breastfeeding reduces the risk of ovarian and breast cancer, heart disease and type 2 diabetes for the mother.

The few things that affect milk production are stress, ineffective latch, not nursing enough and certain medications if the mother and baby are not suffering from any other medical conditions.

However, breastfeeding or formula feeding is a personal choice and there is no judgement on that. The mother gets to decide what's convenient for her and what's best for her baby. Some women experience engorged breasts, cracked nipples and insufficient milk supply and end up switching to bottle feed. Whatever you do is your choice and there's absolutely no judgement or shame.

I started a routine of doing Zumba in the evenings. Even 5 minutes felt like forever. On some days I'd practice my old dance items. Something light like a Padam or Śabdam which comprises more of Abhinaya and less Nritta. The easiest items also make me feel like we are stuck in time. I'd feel breathless and dehydrated as if I was going to faint any minute. But I was surprised that my body was still flexible. I could do the stretches, sit-ups and hip openers like the butterfly exercise without much difficulty. I tried to hold the full squat (Indian toilet) position for a few seconds, I did a few sets of Muzhumandi sit-ups (the dance position of full squatting with heels up), I tried the duck walk every day to make sure my lower abdomen, pelvis and hips were strengthened enough to push a full grown baby out. Even the thought of pushing a human out of my vagina horrified me. The thought of an episiotomy made the nerves from my feet numb. There were nights when the fear of labour did not allow me to sleep peacefully. But as we heard in the series Inventing Anna *"People squat on fields every day. There's nothing special about it."* Yes, people of all races and ethnicities do it. People have done it in the past millions of years ago and continue to do it and will do it a hundred years from now too. Women give birth in hospitals, in the comfort of their homes and even on the fields. Birth is a normal procedure. Cats and dogs do it. It is really as simple as that.

BABY'S POSITION

The ideal position for a vaginal delivery is when the baby's head is downward. This is called the vertex position. Anytime after about 36 weeks, the baby's head starts to descend into the lower part of the uterus and further into the pelvis as the body prepares for labour. The baby's head is considered fixed or engaged when the bi-parietal diameter - the widest part of the head, enters the pelvis. When this happens, your body may show a few symptoms like a lowered baby bump, increased urge to pass urine, discomfort in the pelvic area, back pain, improved breathing etc. Some may feel the baby dropping while others may not even notice this. Baby dropping does not mean labour is induced. It may still take one or two weeks to get the baby out.

A baby is said to be in a breech position when they are positioned feet or bottom towards the opening of the uterus. Most breech babies turn into a head-first position by 36 weeks but some may not. Some breech babies can be born vaginally but in most cases, a C-section is recommended.

There are several types of breech positions:

- Frank breech is when the baby's buttocks are aimed at the vaginal canal with its legs sticking straight up in front of its body.
- The complete breech is when the baby's buttocks are pointing downward and the hips and knees are flexed.
- The footling breech is when one or both of the baby's feet point downward to deliver before the rest of the body.
- The transverse lie is a position where the baby is lying in a horizontal position across your uterus. This would make the shoulder enter the vagina first.

Though a breech baby may be difficult to be delivered vaginally, they can be born perfectly healthy although we can't rule out the possibility of certain birth defects.

You may feel the baby's movements in different areas indicating whether the baby is in vertex or breech position. Your healthcare provider can assess this by feeling your belly or doing an ultrasound to confirm the position.

Though there is no specific reason for the baby to be in a breech position, some factors could contribute to this outcome:

- If you're expecting twins or more
- If there is too much or too little amniotic fluid
- If the uterus is not normal in shape
- If you have fibroids
- If you're suffering from a condition called Placenta Previa - that is when the placenta covers all or part of the cervix

- **If the baby is preterm or if the baby has a birth defect which does not allow it to turn head-down**

In some cases, the doctor can manually flip the baby into a head-down position. The most common method to do this is called External Cephalic Version (EVC). This method is 65% effective and carries some risk. This procedure is performed in the hospital in case of emergencies. The doctor places hands on the abdomen and applies pressure to turn the baby's head down while it is still in the uterus. But sometimes this procedure could aggravate the complications so the option they give you might be a planned C-section.

There is nothing scientifically proven to help you prevent a breech position baby but a few exercises like holding the bridge position or child pose, walking, mild dancing etc. may help.

As we were getting closer to our delivery date, we got our traditional wooden cradle transported from my Valyamma's place in Trissur. Daksh, Trishala and Vyom - Samyuktha's and Sanghamithra's children, were the last ones cradled in it.

It's the family's legacy to keep passing on the cradle generation after generation. This antique baby cradle has put me, my mother, my grandmother, my great-grandfather and many to sleep. We don't know since when it exists. It is also known that the great King Swāthi Thirunāl, Mahārāja of Travancore was born in the same palace from where my great grandfather, Kochappan Thamburān hails - Lakṣmīpuram Palace, Changanāśśery. The palace was built in 1811 AD by Travancore ruler Mahārāni Āyilyam Thirunāl Gauri Lakṣmi Bhāi. It was the palace that gifted many Koi Thampurāns who were illustrious writers and artists such as Rāja Rāja Varma, Kerala Varma Valiya Koi Thampuran, A. R. Rāja Rāja Varma (Also known as Kerala Pānini after his literary achievements) and the musician L. P. R. Varma. History remains a mystery of who all were cradled in this antique "Thoṭṭil" and we can't wait to hang this wooden fortune in our home.

"Omana Thiñgal Kidāvo..." A beautiful composition written by Iriyamman Thampi on the birth of Mahārāja Swāthi Thirunāl Rāma Varma still remains one of the greatest lullabies of all time. Swāthi Thirunāl is considered a brilliant musician and is credited with more than four hundred classical compositions in both Carnatic and Hindustāni styles. The future is promised to no one, but the artistic lineage runs in our family and we never know what our little ray of sunshine would turn out to be...

NUCHAL CORD

An umbilical cord is a lifeline for the baby in the womb. Running from the baby's abdomen to the placenta, the umbilical cord is 50-60 cm long and contains three blood vessels - a vein and two arteries. It provides oxygen, blood and nutrients to the foetus. Normally it lies freely in the amniotic fluid but in some cases, it can get wrapped around the baby's neck. This is called the Nuchal cord or Cord-Around-the Neck (CAN). It could be wrapped once, twice or even thrice. This is a common condition and mostly involves no risks. A 2018 study of obstetrics and gynaecology said that 20-30% of deliveries involve a nuchal cord and the majority of the time babies do just fine after this condition. There are no ways to prevent this as it is caused by random movements of the baby in the womb. Foetal heart rate is constantly monitored during labour. Sometimes the umbilical cord around the neck may get too tight as the baby descends through the vaginal canal causing a reduction in the blood/oxygen supply to the baby which results in a drop of foetal heart rate. This is the reason why many women with a nuchal cord go into an emergency C-section. In many cases, women can deliver vaginally despite a nuchal chord.

CESARIAN BIRTH

A C-section delivery is a surgical procedure performed to deliver a baby when a vaginal birth cannot be done safely. It can be planned ahead of time or performed in an emergency. Sometimes it carries more risks than a normal delivery and requires more rest for recovery.

There could be multiple reasons for undergoing a C-section. Reasons for a planned C-section could be:

- Cephalopelvic Disproportion (CPD) is a condition where the baby's head or body is too large to pass through your pelvis or your pelvis is too small to deliver an average-sized baby.
- Previous C-sections may put you at risk of a uterine rupture and hence the next delivery recommended is most likely to be a C-section. In some cases, women are able to deliver vaginally even after a C-section.
- Transverse lie or Breech positions may make it difficult for vaginal delivery.
- Health conditions like heart disease or genital herpes at the time of delivery may require a C-section.

- Obstructions such as a large uterine fibroid, a pelvic fracture in the past or if you're expecting a baby with certain congenital anomalies may turn out to be the reasons for a planned C-section.

However, sometimes, you may undergo an emergency C-section. The reasons for this could be:

- Foetal distress (irregular heart rate during labour)
- Placental abruption (When the placenta separates from the wall of the uterus before the baby is born.
- Umbilical cord prolapse - When the umbilical cord comes out of the cervix before the baby does.
- Umbilical cord compression
- Prolonged labour - When labour isn't progressing due to several reasons. The cervix may not be dilating, when the cervix doesn't efface or when the baby stops moving down the birth canal

Most planned C-sections are performed using an epidural so you will be wide awake for the delivery. However, in some cases, you may be given general anaesthesia.

A typical C-section takes about 45 minutes from start to finish. The obstetrician will make an incision through your skin into the wall of the abdomen and then cut 3-4 inches into the wall of the uterus. It can be transverse or vertical. The baby is removed, the umbilical cord is cut, the placenta is removed and the incisions are closed with stitches and staples.

Like any surgery, there are risks involved in a cesarean delivery like infections, haemorrhage, a cut that may weaken the uterine wall, abnormalities of the placenta in future pregnancies, foetal injury etc. The recovery from a C-section is more difficult than a normal delivery. You may experience chronic pain and may have trouble for breastfeeding. Pain medications are given when the effect of anaesthesia wears off.

There are risks involved in cesarean or vaginal birth options and the pain one endures for childbirth is inevitable. Trust your healthcare provider and choose the option that is the safest for you and your baby.

Finally, on the 5th of July, I was supposed to go for a check-up. There were no symptoms or signs till the previous night. But when I woke up in the morning and saw my reflection in the mirror, I suddenly felt that my perfectly rounded belly looked like it had fallen. It looks like it's sagging down. Chechi and Amma said that's a sign that the uterus has started its preparation to push the baby out. Maybe this is called the "Baby dropping"!

I wanted to look pretty when I clicked labour room pictures with my newborn or if someone visited me on the second day after delivery like the models we see in baby soap commercials. So I rushed to the parlour to get my eyebrows and waxing done before heading to the hospital, though my dad kept making fun of me. My bags were packed so there was nothing to worry about.

The doctor examined me and said that she could admit me and give me a pain-inducing medicine that would help in opening the cervix. Anxiety kicked in and I had no idea how this was going to be. I kept telling myself it was going to be as easy as a movie shoot.

Scene one - Getting admitted to the hospital

Scene two - Labour room and giving birth

Scene three - Moments with the baby

Scene four - Getting discharged

That's how simple it's going to be.

But my heart kept pounding!

Nithesh had blocked two rooms so that Amma or Mummy could stay in one and he could stay with me. Or if there were too many visitors, we could still have more space.

I took a tablet after dinner and one at 3 AM. Around 4 AM I started getting cramps like I was about to get my periods. By 6 AM it was like a strong menstrual pain and they shifted me to the labour room. The environment was terrifying. I had opted for a private birthing suite. The tainted glass did not allow me to see past it but I could hear screams from other women, I could see nurses running around and hear cluttering of the medical equipments in the tray. The screams and shouting would grow fierce and then soon a baby's cry would be heard. This cycle kept repeating several times. There were so many women who were due on that day I guess. Or was this how a normal day in the gynaecology department looked like? No wonder we are one of the most populated countries in the world.

A junior doctor examined me and said I was 1 cm dilated. They gave me an enema to clear up my stomach and after an hour I was 3 cm dilated. The time was past 7 AM. The nurse on duty was finishing her shift. I held her hand tight like I desperately needed her by my side. But the nurse on the next shift was even more kinder and loving. Ashly stayed by my side throughout the whole procedure. When I started crying, she told me "Chechi, I'm not even married. You all should inspire me to get married and have babies." I smiled and she said she's never seen someone who cries with a smile.

By 9 AM, the pain was unbearable and the abdomen kept changing its shape, protruding on the sides due to the contractions. My favourite nurse Reshma and my godmother gynie arrived. It was a relief to see familiar faces. They examined me and called for an epidural. The anaesthesia doctors were really warm and the epidural worked like abracadabra. The anesthesiologist told me to note the next three contractions. One would be severe, the second would be mild and the third would be painless. Voila! My face brightened and the smile reappeared on my face. I slowly released my fist which was clenching Ashly's hands tight. She assured me that it was all going to be a cakewalk now.

Dr. Susan checked my cervix once again and manually broke my water. I felt like a river was flowing down there. By 10 AM, my mother visited me. She burst out crying seeing me in the blue hospital gown with several devices plugged on me - CTG machine, pulse oximeter, blood pressure etc. I felt better seeing Amma.

By 10.30 AM, the doctor checked me and said I was fully dilated by 10 cm and we were at the final stage of labour. I was frenzied by hysteria. The room suddenly lit up with more lights and everyone scrubbed in. No wonder they call it theatre; the birthing suite lit up like there's a movie shoot going to happen now. I could hear them as if they were meddling with steel cutleries. The doctor then called my husband in. I didn't want to look at his face as I'd get more conscious of myself. I know it wasn't a beautiful sight to see his wife in a pool of blood in an OT. I kept my eyes closed. By 11 AM, I was asked to push. I honestly did not believe a baby could pass through my vagina but I started to push. Without screaming, without crying, I kept pushing in a state of trance by totally surrendering to God. I knew that years of dancing was definitely going to pay me off at this point.

My pelvic floor is stronger than I think it is. I can do this.

I don't know who all were holding my hands, but I surely felt a lot of warmth and support. I still kept my eyes closed and tried to push with a calm, focused mind. Reshma, the head nurse was pushing my abdomen downward to help me.

With the third contraction and push at 11.16 AM, I could feel a tiny human pop out and they put her on my chest for skin-to-skin contact. My eyes welled up as I held her tight.

“It’s a baby girl,” said the doctor. I was really surprised. I never expected it to be a girl though I completely hoped for the same.

I then turned to look at my husband who was patting my shoulder. “*We did it, we created this miracle from scratch*” That’s what our eyes communicated.

And just like that, our entire world changed forever. That’s how our little bundle of happiness, Dheemahee Nithesh Nair was born.

Dheemahee means wise and intelligent. It is a prominent word in all Gāyatrī mantras - Gaṇeśa Gāyatrī, Sūrya Gāyatrī, Santhāna Gopāla Gāyatrī…

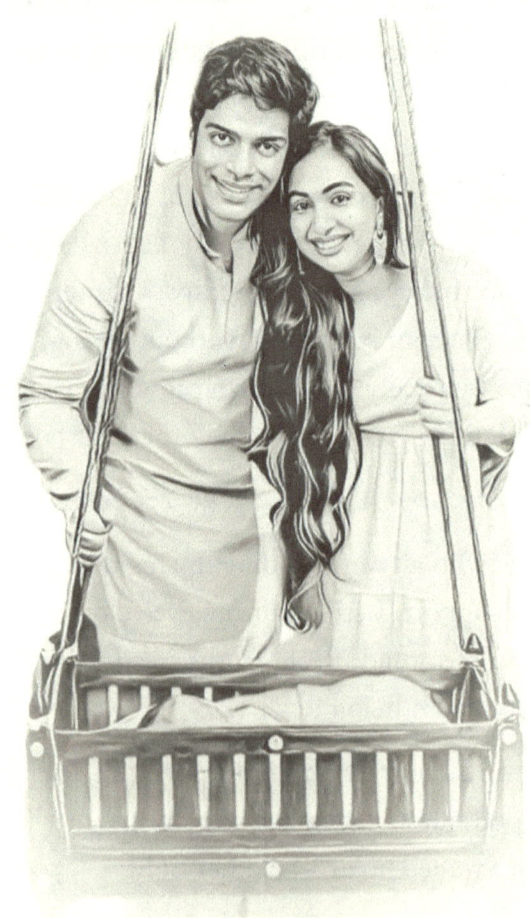

SANTHĀNA GOPĀLA MANTHRA -

Devaki Nandana Govindā

Vāsudeva Jagatpathim

Dehime Thanayam Kṛṣṇahā

Thvāmaham Śaranam Gathām

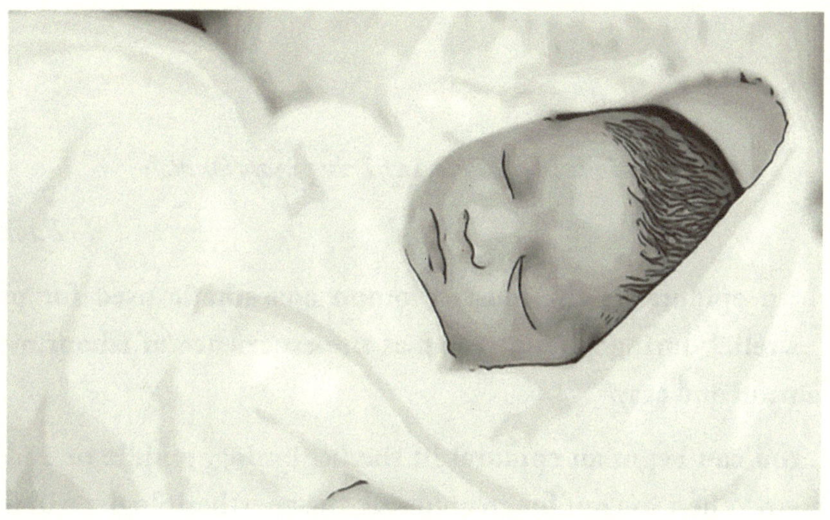

EPIDURAL

"Pain is inevitable, suffering is optional."

– Buddha

An epidural is the most common anaesthetic used for pain relief during labour. It makes the experience of labour more beautiful and easy.

You can begin an epidural in the beginning, middle or end of labour. When you opt for an epidural, the anesthesiologist will first numb the area in your lower back using a local anaesthetic. This makes the procedure painless. The doctor will then insert a needle and a catheter into your lower spine. Some may feel pressure when the needle is inserted. The needle will be removed and the catheter will remain in place for continuous flow of medication. This process takes about five to ten minutes and the results are very quick.

An epidural's job is to block nerve signals responsible for feelings of pain from your belly button to the legs. A urinary tube is inserted in the patient as some may feel numbness in the legs which makes it difficult for them to walk to the toilet. This tube will be removed once the numbness wears off.

Epidural is commonly used during labour but they are also used for surgical procedures in the lower abdomen, pelvis and legs. Hence a patient who opted for an epidural considering normal delivery can use the same anaesthetic if she goes into an emergency C-section.

Epidural allows the mother to relax and rest so that she gains enough strength to push the baby. Epidurals result in positive birth experiences and a 2014 study claims that they result in reducing postpartum depression.

However, there are certain cons associated with this medication. Your blood pressure may drop. Hence oxygen and IV fluid are given to the patient and BP is constantly monitored. Some may feel itchiness but this will go away once the catheter for epidural is removed. The lower back may be sore due to the numbness of the medicine for a few days but there is no evidence proven that permanent back pain is associated with epidurals. Very rarely patients get headaches due to leakage in spinal fluid. But doctors give other medication and it is usually resolved in a few days. If the anesthesiologist is inexperienced or unprofessional - in extremely rare cases - there are chances for permanent nerve damage if the needle or catheter damages the spinal cord or if the epidural area gets unnecessary bleeding or is in contact with infections. However, the risk of permanent damage is extremely low.

Epidurals are generally considered safe but always do your research to understand more about their pros and cons and discuss with your doctor to finalise your plan before the due date. Choosing an epidural or not should be a personal choice, not your family's, not your husband's. It is your body and it should be your choice.

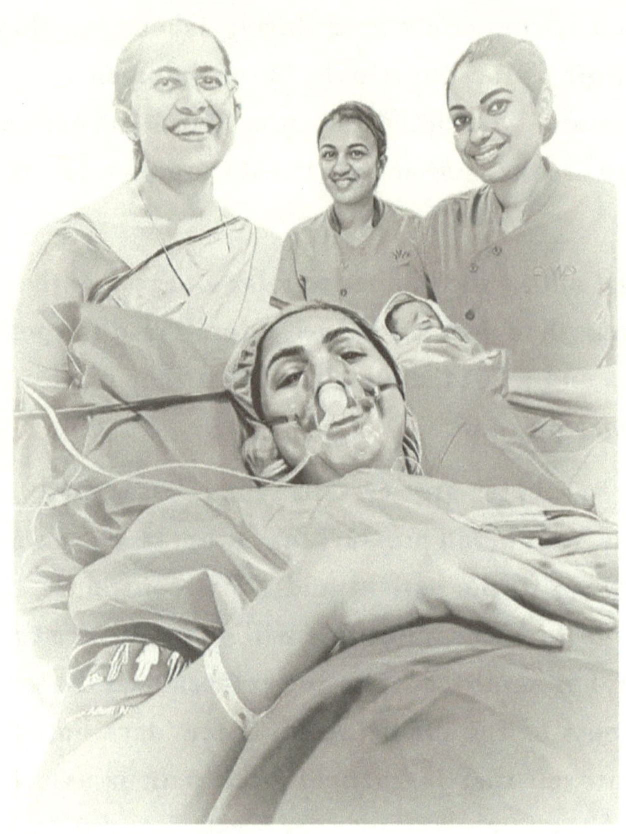

In the end, when everything worked out just miraculously more beautiful than the dread I had, I didn't know whom to thank. Was it the endless prayers by me and my family that began nine months back? Was it the immense support given by my loved ones? Was it the doctor who seemed like God in front of me? Or was it the nurses who were like angels who descended to the earth? Was it years of dancing that helped me with a strong pelvic floor that made me deliver in less than fifteen minutes? Or was it all a combination of a universal blessing? I don't know. I'm only grateful for having all the amazing people by my side. I can't recommend my doctor and the hospital enough for making me so comfortable. Dr. Susan John (OB-GYN), who patiently answered all my doubts for nine months. Her pleasant smiling face was so calming. We meet every month for hardly five minutes, but in those five minutes, I cherish every single second. I know how valuable those five minutes are. She made me so relieved and confident about my entire birth process. Head nurse Reshma who took a special effort in comforting me in every possible way. I'm forever thankful to her. Lekha Aunty, who helped us with consultations and arrangements without having to wait. Dr. Raghu who owns the hospital - Ernakulam Medical Centre, Department of Neonatology, Dr. Grace and all other nurses and PROs, thank you for making my experience of welcoming my little heart so beautiful and hassle-free.

POSTPARTUM

"The grand adventure is about to begin"

– Winnie the Pooh!

WELCOME TO MOTHERHOOD!

The fourth trimester that no one talks about is the postpartum period. Though it is the most beautiful phase of one's life it can be excruciating and exhausting. The mother has not only delivered a baby, but she has also delivered an organ - the placenta. Postpartum is the period from birth to about a couple of months and it can be divided into three phases - acute phase, subacute phase and delayed phase. The WHO describes the postnatal period as the most critical and yet most neglected phase of a woman's life and the shocking part is that most maternal and newborn deaths occur during this period.

The acute phase is the first few hours after giving birth. This is monitored by medical professionals as complications are likely to arise. The newborn takes its first breath about 10 seconds within the delivery. The WHO recommends skin-to-skin contact to establish bonding and regulate the baby's temperature.

The subacute period can last up to six weeks. This is the period where the uterus shrinks to its normal size. 80% of women report at least one health condition during this period and urinary incontinence is a common problem in many. The discharge from the uterus is called lochia and may last till about 4-6 weeks. Stool softeners are given since constipation can be a main issue and the healing sutures can be painful. Some women may feel uterine contractions even after delivery. The cramping is the compression of blood vessels in the uterus to prevent bleeding. Breastfeeding difficulties may arise at this point. Due to the maternal sleep being compromised and rapid hormonal changes in the body, the mother may experience psychological disorders. 80% of women experience postpartum depression and 20% may go into clinical depression. Women with medical/psychiatric conditions like diabetes, hypertension, thyroid etc. should continue to follow up with their primary care provider.

A delayed postpartum period can last up to six months or one year. During this time, muscles and organs return to their pre-pregnancy state. Postpartum alopecia (Hair loss) can occur in some women due to the drop in estrogen levels. But don't worry, it is temporary. 31% of women report long-term health problems during this period.

It is important to give yourself enough care and comfort during this period like how you managed during those nine months. Pregnancy care does not end at the delivery table. This is where the support of your loved ones is needed. The husband, parents, siblings, friends anyone who can support you mentally, physically and financially are important at this point. Don't be afraid to ask for help and don't hesitate to set boundaries with anyone who makes you uncomfortable. Toxic family members add fire to postpartum psychosis. Postpartum counselling and therapy would help you to understand yourself better even if you have family and friends around.

Postnatal Āyurvedic massages and treatments are a necessity for the new mother. Proper nutrition is required for speedy recovery. Get enough sleep, though it sounds impossible with a newborn. A newborn typically sleeps for 16-18 hours a day. You can surely manage some naps during that time, you superwoman! Your body is pure magic. You would have already realised that. How fast did the uterus grow four times its size and how fast did it shrink back to its original size? How fast did melasma cover the entire tummy making it appear dark and ugly and how fast did it all fade away? The recovery is so beautiful and quick. Don't hate your body for simply going from size XS (Extra Small) to M (Medium) or M to L (Large). It has created a human being from scratch, a job that no artificial intelligence is capable of doing. Be proud of yourself. A normal body can endure only 49 units of pain but during childbirth, a woman goes through 57 units of pain. You are stronger than you think you are. Reward yourself for what you have created, rebuild your strength and reclaim your body. Love is the best medicine, so love your body and take that speedy elevator to recovery!

ACKNOWLEDGMENTS

My heartfelt gratitude and sincere thanks to the following people who contributed to my writing.

Dr. Susan John. Thank you for clearing my doubts and vetting this book. You were so positive and encouraging towards my approach to this book. It gave me a lot of confidence.

Ann John, my neighbour and my English teacher who took the effort to edit my first draft. Thank you, Aunty.

My father, A R Unni who has inspired me to write since my childhood. I'm always in awe of your linguistic skills. Love you.

My mother, Urmila Unni who was the only person who believed in my writing. She writes beautifully in Malayalam. Thank you for believing in me Amma.

My husband, Nithesh S Nair who is a constant support to all my endeavours. Thank you for pushing me beyond my comfort zone and teaching me to never settle for anything less than what I deserve.

Hariprasad Varma, yoga therapist. Thank you for giving me the right guidance on prenatal yoga.

Dr. Parvathy Arun and Dr. Krishnaprasad. Thank you for educating me on Ayurveda.

Thanks to all my dance Gurus for teaching me this divine art form Bharatanatyam.

Thank you, Namrata, for helping me to transliterate the Sanskrit words in this book.

Thank you, Photolab, for the illustrations.

Thank you, Shilpa Singh, Doodlabad for the wonderful cover design for the book.

Thank you, Notion Press, for providing me with a platform to publish my first book. Thank you for all the guidance.

Thank you, Dr. C.G. Raghu, for your valuable feedback on this book.

Last but not the least, my Instagram/Facebook friends and followers. Without you all, this book would have never happened. Sometimes a simple comment can uplift a person's confidence. My deepest gratitude to everyone who has touched my path and made me believe that I can write. I hope I did not disappoint you.

BIBLIOGRAPHY

Dr. Ibrahim H Baltagi, Professor at Lebanese American University - Unicef study on brain development

Rujuta Diwekar - Nutrition for each trimester - Pregnancy Notes

Kareen Kapoor Khan - Pregnancy Bible

Dr. P Girija - Jeevani - Ayurveda for women

Dr. Anjali Kumar, Gynaecologist - Maitri vlog

Dr. Fenning - Penn Medicine

Devdutt Pattanaik - Mothers in Hindu mythology - Devlok 2

Nandini Krishna - Cow/Snake - The sacred animals of India

www.ohbabynutrition.com

www.healthline.com

www.lovemajka.com

www.mayoclinic.org

www.webmd.com

www.womenshealth.gov

www.whattoexpect.com

Mylo pregnancy tracker app

https://pjnsbvjournals.com

www.yogamdniy.nic.in

www.clevelandclinic.org

www.americanpregnancy.org

www.dremeilkamel.com - Weekly developments of the foetus

Dr. Alexander Jacob IPS - The Nāgas

Dr. Swathi H V - Care Hospitals - Placenta

www.who.int - Brain Development

www.ingramcontent.com/pod-product-compliance
Lightning Source LLC
LaVergne TN
LVHW091313150826
845673LV00006B/1634

* 9 7 9 8 8 9 2 3 3 7 7 7 9 *